ADVANCE PRAISE FOR *CARING FOR AUTISM*

"A comprehensive, insightful, intimate, and personal guidebook on autism. This book reads like a novel, and you will never want to put it down as you learn about autism diagnosis, prevention, understanding, and treatments from the perspective of a family coping with autism. The author's understanding on autism comes from both professional and personal experience. Whether you are a new parent to autism or a seasoned parent, you will access a step-by-step process from diagnosis to adulthood planning. This is a highly recommended resource from a truly gifted professional that proves to be an abundance of information of ideas, answers, and perspectives to all parents, family members, and practitioners of persons on the autism spectrum. A must read!"

—**Denise Camp Henry, MEd, CCC-SLP**, Private
Speech-Language Pathologist, Columbus, GA

"This book serves as a wonderful resource for families having a family member diagnosed with an autism spectrum disorder. Having Dr. Ellis' deep understanding of autism from a clinician's, as well as from a parent's point of view, provides an enriched and unique source. This book is a great collection of important medical information and the emotional support that parents need as they are going through the process of grief after the diagnosis of autism. I will definitely add this book to the resource list I am providing for families caring for a family member diagnosed with an autism spectrum disorder. This book is highly recommended for clinicians providing services for patients diagnosed with autism in order to better understand and be sensitive to the families' emotional journey."

—**Franciska Kocsner, PsyD**, Licensed Clinical Psychologist,
The Brain Center, Columbus, GA

"Dr. Ellis writes from the compassionate heart of a parent yet teaches the many facets of autism on a professional level. An excellent reference for anyone interested in learning more about the complexity of this wide spectrum disability."

—**Melissa Lape EdS**, Parent, Special Education Teacher,
Toccoa, GA

CARING FOR AUTISM

CARING *for* AUTISM

PRACTICAL ADVICE FROM
A PARENT AND PHYSICIAN

❧

MICHAEL A. ELLIS, DO
Clinical Assistant Professor
Mercer University School of Medicine;
Clinical Associate Professor
Philadelphia College of Osteopathic Medicine (PCOM),
GA Campus;
Medical Director of Child and Adolescent Psychiatry
The Bradley Center, St. Francis Hospital;
Committee on Lifelong Learning for the Academy of Child
and Adolescent Psychiatry (AACAP)
Trustee for Georgia Council on Child
and Adolescent Psychiatry
Columbus, GA

with

LORI LAYTON ELLIS, BS, MPH

OXFORD
UNIVERSITY PRESS

OXFORD
UNIVERSITY PRESS

Oxford University Press is a department of the University of Oxford. It furthers the University's objective of excellence in research, scholarship, and education by publishing worldwide. Oxford is a registered trade mark of Oxford University Press in the UK and certain other countries.

Published in the United States of America by Oxford University Press
198 Madison Avenue, New York, NY 10016, United States of America.

Library of Congress Cataloging-in-Publication Data
Names: Ellis, Michael A., author.
Title: Caring for autism : practical advice from a parent and physician / by Michael A. Ellis, DO, Board Certified Child and Adolescent Psychiatrist, Clinical Assistant Professor, Mercer University School of Medicine, Clinical Associate Professor, Philadelphia College of Osteopathic Medicine (PCOM), GA campus, Medical Director of Child and Adolescent Psychiatry, The Bradley Center, St. Francis Hospital, Columbus, GA.
Description: New York, NY : Oxford University Press, [2018] | Includes bibliographical references and index.
Identifiers: LCCN 2017007788 | ISBN 9780190259358 (alk. paper)
Subjects: LCSH: Autism in children. | Autistic children—Care. | Parents of autistic children.
Classification: LCC RJ506.A9 .E4445 2018 | DDC 618.92/85882—dc23
LC record available at https://lccn.loc.gov/2017007788

1 3 5 7 9 8 6 4 2

Printed by Sheridan Books, Inc., United States of America

To my children Gabby, Lexi, and Zach

Contents

CONTENTS

———

CONTENTS

CONTENTS

CONTENTS

Acknowledgments

The completion of this book could not have been possible without the participation and sacrifice of my wife and family. I would like to express my appreciation to the countless others who reviewed this book and offered advice. I would also like to acknowledge my patients and their families as they have taught me much of what I have learned over the years.

I would especially like to thank my daughter, Gabby, who is my inspiration and greatest teacher. She has helped more people than she will likely ever know by giving me a better and more personal understanding of autism.

I would also like to thank my other two children, Lexi and Zach, who bring me much joy.

And to God, the giver of wisdom and hope, who makes all things possible.

I would especially like to express my appreciation to the following professionals who reviewed sections of this book: to my mentor and friend, Sandra B. Sexson, MD, of The Medical College of Georgia at Augusta University; Hayden Barnes, Esq.; and Carlie Frederick, APRN-BC.

Contributor

————————

Lori Layton Ellis, BS, MPH

Master's in Public Health with focus on Maternal and Child
  Health from Nova Southeastern College of Osteopathic
  Medicine
Bachelor of Science in Microbiology and Cell Science; Minor
  in Education
Co-founder of Chattahoochee Autism Support Group
Mother of child with Autism Spectrum Disorder
Columbus, GA

CARING FOR AUTISM

A FATHER'S PERSPECTIVE
ON AUTISM

A father has a unique perspective on autism and its impact on his family. I write about my experience as a father of a child with autism as it is fairly typical in terms of the timing of concerns and the dilemmas faced during the process of a child's diagnosis with autism (autism spectrum disorder). It is important that fathers know what is "normal" to feel and think about ASD and about their child, in general. Knowing that you are not the only one with your experience and feelings helps you not to feel alone. This by itself can be therapeutic.

The diagnosis of ASD is arguably the worst diagnosis that a child psychiatrist can give a young child. It is also the most devastating diagnosis that one can give to the family. Before the official diagnosis of my daughter, at about 2½ years of age, my wife had expressed concern a couple of times regarding my daughter's limited speech. I thought my wife was overreacting and being a "worrywart." Although I acknowledged that my daughter's speech was a little behind, I simply thought that she was going to catch up. "Children develop at their own pace," I thought. However, when she had only a few words at 24 months, I knew this was not "normal." In fact, our pediatrician, who we saw only at our daughter's monthly checkups, had never noticed any abnormalities in our child until we finally expressed concern regarding her speech delay. She referred us to a speech therapist at our strong request.

On some level, we probably knew something was wrong. My wife had actually mentioned the word autism once, but I do not think we actually thought that this was going to be her diagnosis. My wife and I knew very little about ASD, but we knew enough to be concerned that she seemed to enjoy being by herself too much, had a speech delay, and had limited eye contact. These symptoms are very typically the first symptoms noticed by parents, alerting them to a problem. That was us. She also had tantrums, but we simply assumed this was the "terrible two's." As she was our first child, we did not know how challenging a young child's behavior was supposed to get.

At about the same time, I had just applied to a child and adolescent psychiatry fellowship program and was completing my last year of adult psychiatry residency when we realized that my daughter might have ASD. I was not yet trained in child psychiatry, and I really did not know much about autism or typical development.

MY CHILD'S DIAGNOSIS

When we attended my daughter's first speech therapy evaluation, the speech therapist immediately told my wife that she thought my daughter had autism. Our pediatrician had never diagnosed ASD in my child nor had she alluded to any problem like this. My wife and I were distraught. "How dare the speech therapist give this diagnosis!" we thought. She was not qualified to give this diagnosis and even her mentioning "autism" seemed irresponsible.

This informal diagnosis sent us into a tailspin. This was our first child and she was supposed to be "perfect." We had planned on having children for years. All of our dreams and hopes for our child came crashing down. Our denial was shattered.

Making the diagnosis more overwhelming was the lack of guidance in what steps we were to take next. At first, there was really no one to help decide upon a treatment plan or to give us even a rough prognosis. Even the autism resources of which we were aware proved to be scattered or not available in our area. We felt lost. For months, we continued speech therapy while waiting to get in with a developmental pediatrician as recommended by our speech therapist. Once we had our initial evaluation by the developmental pediatrician, my daughter received an official autism diagnosis and was referred to occupational therapy to help with fine motor skills deficits and to "learn to play" appropriately. Although the developmental pediatrician was experienced, she was the only one in town and as a result had a long waiting list of 6 months for both initial and follow-up appointments. There also was not a behavioral therapist (Board Certified Behavior Analyst [BCBA]) available in our area—not that we even knew what this was at the time. This therapy of Applied Behavioral Analysis (ABA) is now known to be the most evidence-based treatment for ASD. I would not know much about ABA for another 2 to 3 years.

We continued the above therapies of occupational therapy and speech therapy with some small successes. We still felt helpless, and our vague treatment strategy seemed nearly hopeless. I wanted to fight this disorder and do whatever I could, but I had no idea how to help. I was in denial at first and then this changed to sadness and self-doubt: I could not believe that I had not noticed the signs of ASD earlier. It was quite humbling. I was also angry and frustrated that our pediatrician had not diagnosed autism earlier and before anyone else. I was confused.

WHY DID THIS HAPPEN TO MY CHILD?

What had we done wrong? My wife and I were overly cautious during pregnancy regarding what she ate and which products she used. She refused any medications, including over-the-counter medications such as Tylenol. She refused to consume any caffeine, chocolate, or even peanut butter. She used as little personal products as possible and would not dye or color her hair. She ate plenty of fruits and vegetables. We even laughed when she was pregnant at how "overboard" she was going in order to have the perfect baby.

After I determined that we could not have done anything wrong during the pregnancy, I thought we must have done something wrong after the delivery. Did we not interact with her enough? Did she watch too much television? Was it my fault genetically? Every question that you can imagine came to my mind. No one in my family had ASD. I just could not understand. My wife blamed herself more than I did, and she questioned everything she had done. It was hard to comfort her and convince her that she had not done anything wrong.

As the father, "I am supposed to protect my family and child," I thought. However, clearly I could not protect my daughter. As fathers do, I just wanted to "fix" it. As a doctor, it is my job to diagnosis and cure illnesses. I was powerless to do this. I often thought, "I'd rather have this illness myself." I wanted to take it away from my daughter. I also could not imagine how I could watch my child struggle through this for the rest of her life. I could not calmly wait 10 to 20 years to know what the outcome of this disorder would be. I worried constantly. Her ASD seemed to be never-ending grief and worry for us. Even though

I loved my daughter more than anything, I found myself wanting to pull away and immerse myself in my work. This was so that I could escape the difficult situation and find a way to cope, but also because I wanted to feel competent and "good" at something. It was not possible for me to feel even adequate as a father because it seemed as if there was little that I could do. I also had unexplainable guilt and wanted to spoil her to alleviate this guilt.

Later, I was angry with God. I was angry that He could do this to me, to my family, and especially to my daughter. Her diagnosis of ASD challenged my worldview and perspective on life. I thought, "How could God let this happen to innocent, helpless children?" It felt too cruel. I was also concerned that if this could happen to my daughter, with no family history of ASD, then this could happen to any child. This fact, combined with the rapidly increasing prevalence of ASD, made me wonder why more people were not concerned or addressing this apparent autism epidemic.

As the years have passed, the pain of ASD has lessened. I found medications to help my daughter with her tantrums and concentration, and I discovered the very helpful therapy of ABA. My daughter improved slowly over the years, and she has largely exceeded my expectations. Acceptance of my daughter's ASD has come, providing some peace. My family has established a "new normal." I have learned to love and appreciate my daughter for who she is as her own unique person. She provides me with daily laughter and joy. While always difficult and unpredictable, it does get better.

LESSONS LEARNED

There are numerous points to note from my story. First, unfortunately the ASD diagnosis is not uncommonly missed by pediatricians and other professionals. Sometimes this is due to inexperience or lack of training, while at other times it is due to the very quick nature of current primary care physician visits. This is due, at least in part, to the low reimbursement rates by insurance companies, who have come to dictate just about everything in healthcare. These visits are too short to pick up on more subtle ASD symptoms. Furthermore, in some cases of ASD, the diagnosis is not as obvious at a very young age. Many times it is indeed first the teacher, parent, or another professional (speech therapist) who expresses concern for possible ASD.

Second, anger and denial are very common during the initial diagnostic process. There is also a prolonged grief that the parent experiences that may even last a lifetime. Many of the traditional stages of grief are experienced and these may wax and wane for many years. This grieving process can interfere with appropriate and timely evaluation and treatment. It may cause the parent to delay therapies and avoid medication management considerations. Even more of a problem, the parent who becomes clinically depressed risks further harm to the child by interacting less with the child and not researching the best treatments for the child. This is further compounded by a general lack of guidance by professionals and the fact that the parent must be actively engaged in treatment. Parents must be an advocate for their child in all domains of life, such as therapy, medication management, socialization, and education. Also, as the child's brain is most malleable at a young age, delaying the start of therapy for any reason will affect potential achievements and long-term outcomes. You must not allow denial or grief to interfere with your child getting timely and appropriate treatment.

Third, as a father, you are very important to your family and child. At first you will feel extreme frustration and helplessness in raising your child with ASD. However, your child will have improvements and the grief will lessen over time. Try not to worry too much. Be there for your wife and child. Listen to them. You do not always have to "fix" the problem to make it better.

Listening alone is quite therapeutic. Be an active participant and do not withdraw as an escape. However, try to develop a hobby that provides a well-deserved break. Make sure you have a support system. Consider therapy yourself. If you are not doing well, then neither will your child or family. Some parents may need medication or mental health treatment for themselves due to the severe stress of raising a child with ASD. Do not waste time. Make sure that you research treatments and therapies yourself and engage in the local autism community. Also, do not "reinvent the wheel." Other families in your area will likely have good advice regarding which doctors and therapists are best and which treatments are available and trustworthy. Search for a child psychiatrist or developmental pediatrician who has a sound reputation and experience in dealing with ASD. Not all doctors are equal in this area.

Fourth, you should not blame yourself for your child's autism. We do not know what causes autism in the overwhelming majority of cases (see Chapter 4). Your child needs you to be engaged and hopeful. Do not dwell on the past or worry about your child's future. Take it one day at a time. There is no way to accurately predict your child's future or prognosis. Your child needs you to have acceptance and for you to be a cheerleader for him or her. Develop a support system to help you through the difficult times. ASD can be quite a roller-coaster ride of ups and downs. You need someone to laugh with about the humorous things our children do. You also need someone to cry with in those moments that you feel things are never going to get better. For parents of children who have aggression and tantrums, please know that your child may have seemingly random, cyclic episodes of worsening. However, tell yourself that this severe episode will pass just as it did the last time.

Fifth, consider all of your options in terms of various therapies, medications, educational opportunities, and so forth. Do not be afraid to get an evaluation by a child psychiatrist or developmental pediatrician, speech therapist, occupational therapist, BCBA, psychologist, physical therapist, neurologist, geneticist, and other professionals as needed. If for some reason you do not agree with the treatment recommendations offered by one of these providers, you do not necessarily have to follow it. You will not be trapped into doing something that you do not want to do, but you should discuss openly any reservations with the provider. You might have misconceptions about the proposed treatment that need to be resolved.

Lastly, do not underestimate the importance of social support and faith. Many parents state that they have lost friends because their friends do not know how to help or cannot tolerate the ASD behaviors. If you lose friends, then make new friends who are able to understand your challenges. Do not pull away from society or life in general. Join an autism support group or, if one is not available, create one. This will tremendously help you to not feel alone. Also, a part of the growth process is found in acceptance and "finding meaning." Do not avoid this part of the process. This will take some time but is necessary for your own mental health. Furthermore, religious communities can be a great source of acceptance, understanding, and support as well. Do not be afraid to recognize your anger with God or "life" so that you can deal with it. Express your feelings and do not hold them in. Talk to someone you can trust. It is advisable to talk with a religious leader in your community; he or she may be able to help you find peace.

It is my sincere hope that you will find the following chapters both informative and supportive. The journey on which you are about to embark will be filled with many trials and difficult times. However, this is your child and you can and will see to it that you make things better for your child and your family. There will be not only hard times, but many good times. In the end you will be able to appreciate your child for who he or she is and find a great deal of humor in your life. I love my daughter and often I think that if she did not have autism, I would miss the person she is now. You will feel this way too, if you do not already. Even though your child cannot always (or ever, in some cases) express his or her love for you, he or she does love you in his or her own way. Take comfort in the fact that you are not alone, as millions of other families are struggling with ASD as well. Furthermore, an enormous and ever-increasing amount of research is being done on autism. This should provide you with hope for a better life for you and your child.

2

A MOTHER'S PERSPECTIVE
ON AUTISM

By Lori Layton Ellis, BS, MPH

From the moment you discover that you are going to be a parent, the hopes, dreams, and expectations you have for yourself and your child flood your mind. No matter how your child is to arrive, your heart is full of hope and promise. You begin to let yourself plan your future. Will your child become president, a doctor, a lawyer, work in the family business, or win the Nobel Peace Prize? Will he or she possess a special talent or skill? Your mind wanders and daydreams of all that is to come. The moment they place your beautiful child in your arms, you realize that there is no greater feeling. You are in love. There is no feeling deeper or grander. The unimaginable joy and gratitude for the blessing of your child is overwhelming.

We all know those moments where your heart surged out of your body in awe of the blessing you were given. You may have even asked yourself, "How did I get so lucky?" I can relate. The moment they placed my daughter in my arms for the first time,

I knew I had a greater purpose. I would not find out how much for another two years. I devoted myself to her; her care, her introduction to the world, and to the very amazing person I knew she would become. I gave everything of myself tirelessly to her. Her every whimper, cry, or gesture was met with a response. I could anticipate her needs and wants before she fully expressed them. I thought I had an undeniable bond with my daughter. I did. I had a bond that needed no words. That was the problem: we did not need words.

If you are like me, you noticed at first subtle differences in your child, and then later there were glaring and alarming indications something was not developing correctly. But, no matter your education or your intelligence level, denial can be a powerful thing. It can make you justify and explain away any petty difference or blame another person for his or her audacity to suggest your child is anything but perfect. It can even cause you to isolate yourself from the reality that lies in the outside world. After all, weren't you there to protect your child from the negativities of the world? You begin dreading taking your child out to play groups because she cannot do the things others are doing. But still, you will not let yourself accept it. What do other moms know? All children develop at different rates, right? I can still hear myself saying these words. They haunt me. I lived in this denial for almost a year. I thought I could change the inevitable differences by pretending they did not exist. I could hold on to the dreams I had spun. I did not have to listen to the naysayers. I could continue to be blissfully happy with my "lucky" little life. But I could not, no matter how hard I tried. I thought I would show them. I would make the medical professionals tell me she was fine. I was not going to let anyone say otherwise. But they did: they showed me my dreams were going to have to be redreamed.

At 18 months old my daughter had few to no words. We had our own form of language. I thought my anticipation of her needs was normal, almost superior to other moms. I wondered why other kids needed words so early. We did not. "We must be closer than other parents and children," I thought. Denial is a self-protective coping mechanism. However, it was not healthy: my daughter needed to communicate with others, not just me. Once I opened up my mind to the possibility that she needed others, I began to see the differences. She was not just really smart at reorganizing patterns and shapes, she was using shapes and patterns to calm herself. She did not just like order, she survived off it. She was different. I had to find out what that meant.

The first person to say, "I think your daughter has autism" was a speech pathologist we were sent to for an initial evaluation. I thought, "She has no idea what she is talking about." So she liked to stack books repeatedly in rows. She was too young to read; what else was she supposed to do with them? So she does not make eye contact; she is looking at your mouth to read your lips. "She DOES NOT have autism," I thought. But she did. I immediately resented the woman in that room. She became the focus of my rage. Honestly, I still have a bit of residual feelings about her to this day. I demanded we be sent to a "real" expert. Our journey had begun. We had just embarked on the most difficult, rewarding, and frightening voyage of our lives. Our family of three was about to change, but as I learned after many trials and tribulations, that was "okay."

My daughter did not speak full sentences until she was nearly 4 years old. Even then, she spoke in a very template-like form that was robotic in nature: "I want [insert need], please." It was always the same. ALWAYS. My heart ached for a spontaneous sentence such as, "Hey, look mommy!" or "I love you!" That did not come for some time, but it did come. I am grateful for that. I have found myself a lot more grateful than I once was. I had every reason to be happy and content, but after my daughter's diagnosis with autism, I became so much more thankful for every little gain. I had a new frame of reference. While others found it disheartening that my daughter could not do what others her age could, I was thrilled that she learned her own name and responded to it when called. That moment changed our lives. Every new word she spoke, every time she performed a "typical" behavior, and every day we made it without some sort of tantrum or meltdown due to frustration (on both of our parts) was a day to celebrate. We found a way through the silence. We found a way to move forward. The pace did not matter because we were making progress. We continued to prove that slow and steady DOES win the race.

If you can relate to these moments of joy and disappointment, you are not alone. As parents of children who have ASD, we share so many similar moments and paths. We persevere though our trials with attributes similar to those of a marathon competitor. We start out to win the race with sheer strength and speed, and prepare to finish with determination and endurance. It will take all of what you are "made of" to raise your "special" child. It will teach you more about yourself and your strength than you can imagine. You can complete the race. You can do it with honor, faith, hope, and LOVE. You must give yourself the opportunity to set your own stride. Do not try to follow the lead runners. You cannot compete with them. They do not have the same path. They are not going to take the scenic route that you are going to travel. They will not get to stop and notice all the beauty in the smallest of places: the fresh dew on the grass or the tiniest of creatures lurking beneath the leaves of a century-old oak.

Your path is not about the competition; it is about the completion. You are going to need to rest along the way. You are going to need to ask others for a hand-up and even a tag-out. That is okay. The point is to finish. You need to listen to someone who has begun the race before you. You can do this. It will not always feel like it. In fact, it will often feel like you are not making much progress. It will feel as if you are destined to lose, but you are NOT. You are a hero to your child. You are a hero to your family, and a hero to all of us who have run before you. We know what it takes. We understand your struggles, but we also understand the reward you will find in running with all you are and all you have. There is satisfaction in knowing that our children do not run alone, but with their biggest supporter and fan beside them every step of the way. The more effort you put toward your goal, the more you will hit your winner's stride. We are a community of runners. We stand united with each of you in your path. You will conquer. You will succeed. You are a champion and a force to be reckoned with in the eyes of the child for whom you run. Never lose sight of why you started the race or why you must finish victorious.

We have met with so many challenges in raising our daughter. It has not been easy; in fact, it has been the most difficult task of my life. I stated earlier that my daughter was my purpose. I knew that I was put on this earth to be her mother, and it was going to be my job to see she achieved every goal SHE set forth. I had to learn to let her take the lead and set the pace, but I still run alongside her no matter where she goes. How do I do it? Well, the frank answer is day by day. I do not mean that in the cliché way—I mean literally day to day. I do not make a habit of anticipating where we will be a month from now. Our lives are fluid in the sense of progress and functionality. It takes a lot of patience and a lot of love. Sometimes that love is for the moment not reciprocated in a typically measurable way, but believe me, it is there. It takes immeasurable strength and determination. You have to work on yourself and your environment daily. It is as much a self-evolving journey as it is a journey of courage. You cannot be passive. You cannot be weak. You have to stand tall and be proud. You were chosen to do great things. It may not be painting the Mona Lisa or building the pyramids, but to raise a child with autism has no equal in triumph and accomplishment. It is more difficult than any other task given, but if you truly understand the impact you are having on the world, one child at a time, the outcome is undeniably a great legacy. Do not worry about the naysayers: they do not have the guts, determination, and sheer will that you do. You are a parent with a child with autism. Your superpower has been revealed. As long as you believe in yourself and your child, you can both soar. Different is not less. Different is special.

I wanted to convey a short story that I was told a few years ago that has brought me much hope, strength, and conviction. Although I have not been able to prove it as fact or fiction, the hope and dreams behind the story are real. Albert Einstein is believed to have shown many of the signs and symptoms of autism. He was unable to speak by age 3. One day, it is reported, he brought a note home from school to give only to his mother. She read it aloud and, as the story goes, his mother read, "Your son is a genius and does not have enough good teachers for training him. Please teach him yourself." Einstein's mother homeschooled him from that point forward. Many years later, it was reported that he found the letter hidden away in his mother's things. When he read the letter, it stated, "Your son is addled (mentally ill). We won't let him come back to school anymore." Einstein cried and then wrote in his diary, "Albert Einstein was an addled child that, by a hero mother, became the genius of the century."

We are all capable of being our child's hero. Our children have unique but amazing potentials. I have redreamed many a dream for my daughter, but in the end whatever she becomes is greater than anything I could have imagined because she is who she is meant to be.

ASSESSMENT AND DIAGNOSIS
OF AUTISM SPECTRUM DISORDER

The assessment and diagnosis phase of autism spectrum disorder (ASD) is a very difficult time for the parent. You will likely feel completely bewildered. You will be filled with many mixed emotions such as love for your child and fear for your child's future. You may feel like your heart is breaking. But I can tell you, you are going to make it through this—just like I have. You will likely have to overcome significant denial to even discuss the unusual signs or symptoms that you have noticed in your young child. You may be afraid to hear the term "autism" come from your pediatrician's mouth. However, you are about to start a very important journey with your child. You have to be strong in order to obtain for your child vital treatments and therapies that can dramatically improve your child's life and future.

Theoretically, ASD is not difficult to recognize and diagnose. However, in practice, it can be challenging. The full spectrum of symptoms included in ASD is quite wide. One child may appear quite typical with only minor eccentricities while another has significant intellectual disability, social impairment, self-injurious behavior, and aggression. No two individuals with ASD are exactly alike. In fact, individuals with autism are often more different than similar. We cannot easily pigeonhole or stereotype our children. Further complicating diagnosis, professionals often have little training in ASD, even in fields that have autism within their scope of practice. Furthermore, children with more subtle ASD symptoms or those who are "high-functioning" (more verbal and with more capabilities in general) do not always have symptoms that are evident at a very young age. At times, autism symptoms may not be identifiable until social problems become more significant as the child grows older. Primary care physicians are not typically able to spend long enough with your child during visits to pick up on the sometimes subtle signs needed to alert them to a possible ASD diagnosis. For these reasons, laypeople and professionals from many specialties often struggle to diagnose ASD early.

In practice, I have seen children misdiagnosed with other disorders or even told definitively that their child does not have ASD when it was diagnosed recently by another provider. I have seen children misdiagnosed as having bipolar disorder simply because they have "rages" that were really autism tantrums. I have heard primary care physicians making statements such as, "It can't be autism; he's too smart," "He's too high-functioning," and "He gave me too much eye contact." In regards to a speech delay associated with ASD, I have heard some physicians state, "It will get better on its own." These statements simply indicate lack of experience with the broad spectrum of autism. Often, otherwise competent psychologists and psychiatrists misinterpret ASD symptoms or do not notice them at all. I recommend asking the professional how comfortable he or she is in diagnosing and treating autism if you suspect that your child has ASD.

In this chapter, we will briefly discuss the history of autism. Second, we will discuss the typical presentation of ASD and the clinical signs and symptoms. Third, we will go over the other disorders that can mimic symptoms of ASD. These other disorders or set of problems need to be considered by your treating physician when diagnosing your child with autism; this is called the *differential diagnosis*. Fourth, we will discuss the common comorbid disorders associated with autism. Sometimes, the comorbidities are at least as problematic as the autism. You need to know these because they can be treated with medication and therapies. Fifth, we will discuss the general steps taken to appropriately assess for ASD. This is necessary to know so that you can feel confident that your child has the correct diagnosis and that all proper avenues have been investigated. The more knowledge you have, the better you can understand your child and advocate for him or her.

HISTORY OF AUTISM

The first person to describe autism was Leo Kanner in 1943. He reported on 11 children who had difficulty relating to peers and were sensitive to change. He noted that these children had a marked lack of interest in other people, especially compared to other children. If language did develop, it often presented as echolalia (echoing back what was said to them), and their thoughts were concrete. They often did not pick up on humor and were very literal. Kanner noted that the children had repetitive movements that were unusual and purposeless, called stereotypies (1).

Autism was first believed to be a form of childhood psychosis, but by the 1970s it was found to be a distinctive problem that was not related to psychosis. It was not officially recognized as a diagnosis until 1980 in the third edition of the *Diagnostic and Statistical Manual of Mental Disorders* (DSM-III), the manual used by all medical and mental health professionals to describe and diagnose mental illnesses. By 2000, in the fourth revised edition (DSM-IV-TR), autism was considered one of the pervasive developmental disorders, which also included Rett's disorder, Asperger's disorder, childhood disintegrative disorder, and pervasive developmental disorder not otherwise specified (PDD-NOS) (1). The autism diagnosis required that the child had problems in three domains of functioning—social relatedness, communication/play, and restricted interests—and onset of these symptoms had to be by age 3.

Rett's disorder, Asperger's disorder, childhood disintegrative disorder, and PDD-NOS all have similar presentations to autism, which is why I include this information here. However, should your child be diagnosed with something other than ASD, ask your physician or provider for specific details.

The most recent update to the DSM, the DSM-5, was published in May 2013. In this latest manual, the previous diagnoses of autism, PDD-NOS, and Asperger's disorder were officially combined into the single diagnosis of ASD. You might be familiar with the DSM-5 because it caused a lot of controversy within the autism community. Many were afraid that their child would no longer meet criteria for autism. Others were unhappy that the Asperger's diagnosis was disappearing, as they felt their child with Asperger's disorder was significantly different than those with full autism. In the perception of some, Asperger's disorder was less severe and even carried with it less stigma. Many liked the notion of an Asperger's diagnosis because laypeople at times perceived those with this disorder to be geniuses.

Recent research has shown that the fear that children with previous diagnoses of autism, PDD-NOS, or Asperger's would no longer meet criteria for the new ASD diagnosis is unwarranted. About 91% of children with DSM-IV PDD will retain the diagnosis under the DSM-5 for ASD. Also, the sensitivity (diagnosing autism when it is present) remains high with the new

DSM-5 diagnosis. Specificity (not diagnosing autism when it is not present) is better for DSM-5 diagnosis than DSM-IV, which accomplished the goal of the DSM-5 committee. This will lead to fewer misclassifications, especially avoiding the inappropriate inclusion into the autism spectrum of those with only attention-deficit/hyperactivity disorder (ADHD), intellectual disability, language disorders, or anxiety disorders (2). The DSM-5 changes were made because there was little evidence to support the diagnostic differences between the different DSM-IV-TR PDDs. Based on my experience, I would agree. I do not find the old PDD distinctions helpful diagnostically or in terms of predicting outcomes or prognosis. You should be aware of these changes so that you understand why your child's physician may not use the older and more familiar terms, and so that you do not worry that your child will lose services with the recent changes in diagnosis.

SYMPTOMS OF ASD

According to the DSM-IV, difficulties with social relatedness need to be striking when compared to typically developing peers. For your child to be diagnosed with ASD, he or she should have marked impairment in even nonverbal communication and peer relationships. There should be impairment in social and emotional reciprocity. There may be a total lack of verbal communication without an attempt to compensate through other means of communication. Even if your child is verbal, he or she may have difficulty starting or continuing an appropriate conversation. Your child may also have stereotyped and repetitive language and lack age-appropriate imaginative play. The impairments in interests include circumscribed interests (or encompassing preoccupations), insistence on sameness or nonfunctional routines, repetitive or stereotyped movements/mannerisms, and preoccupation with parts of objects.

For example, when my daughter was in first and second grade, she loved Dora the Explorer. Dora was her circumscribed interest to the exclusion of everything else. She did not want to do anything except watch this TV show or think about Dora all day. She even was interested in peers who looked more like Dora. When a classmate who looked like Dora was absent from school, she would have severe tantrums. Furthermore, she could not tolerate even simple changes in routine, such as changes to the order in which school subjects were taught or the rearrangement of even one desk in the classroom. All of these changes caused devastating tantrums. These stories likely sound very familiar to you, but there are many possible common symptoms that your child with ASD may display. Below is a list of the most common signs and symptoms in those with ASD.

Commonly Seen Signs and Symptoms in Those with ASD
+ Doesn't respond to his or her name by 12 months of age
+ Doesn't point at objects to show interest (point at an airplane flying over) by 14 months
+ Doesn't play "pretend" games (pretend to feed a doll) by 18 months
+ Avoids eye contact and wants to be alone
+ Has trouble understanding other people's feelings or talking about his or her own feelings
+ Has delayed speech and language skills
+ Repeats words or phrases over and over (echolalia)
+ Gives unrelated answers to questions
+ Gets upset by minor changes
+ Has obsessive interests
+ Flaps hands, rocks body, or spins in circles
+ Has unusual reactions to the way things sound, smell, taste, look, or feel

Most often the first sign that alerts the pediatrician or parent to a problem is a language delay or deficits in communication. This may be a delay in language compared to other peers, a lack of language, or the abnormal use of language. Typically, a child who may have autism presents with signs and symptoms between 18 to 24 months. But remember, not all signs are the same in each child. Sometimes, a child may have language that is not functional but contains a lot of echolalia, the simple repetition of heard words. Other children with ASD may not have a language delay but may speak tangentially and only about their own circumscribed interests without noticing that the listener may have stopped listening. They may speak in a monotone or have unusual inflections. Sometimes their voices can sound robotic (3). Below is a list of red flags regarding communication that will alert you and your provider to further investigate a possible ASD diagnosis (4).

Red Flags Related to Communication
+ Delayed speech and language skills
+ Repeats words or phrases over and over (echolalia)
+ Reverses pronouns (e.g., says "you" instead of "I")
+ Gives unrelated answers to questions
+ Does not point or respond to pointing
+ Uses few or no gestures (e.g., does not wave goodbye)
+ Talks in a flat, robot-like, or sing-song voice
+ Does not pretend in play (e.g., does not pretend to feed a doll)
+ Does not understand jokes, sarcasm, or teasing

You, as a parent, may notice less eye contact than would be expected in your infant or toddler. This may go unrecognized for some time if this is your first child. Also, if your child has significant ADHD symptoms, you might explain away his or her poor eye contact as "my child just won't pay attention or sit still long enough to look at me." When looking at a person's face, your child may look at the person's mouth and not his or her eyes.

Children with ASD also have a level of abnormal social reciprocity. This is often described as the "give and take" during social interactions and also requires the child to take another person's perspective. "Normal" interaction between children is clearly impaired in those with ASD: they have difficulty reading body language, responding to nonverbal cues, and maintaining joint attention (ability to attend to an activity with another person), which is why they are socially awkward. A well-known red flag is the inability to point to an object to show interest at 18 months. A typical child should be able to point to bring something to the attention of the caregiver. Below is a list of differences in social skills that you may notice in your child.

Red Flags Related to Social Skills
+ Does not respond to name by 12 months of age
+ Avoids eye contact
+ Prefers to play alone
+ Does not share interests with others
+ Interacts only to achieve a desired goal
+ Has flat or inappropriate facial expressions
+ Does not understand personal space boundaries
+ Avoids or resists physical contact
+ Is not comforted by others during distress
+ Has trouble understanding other people's feelings or talking about his or her own feelings

Another telltale sign that your child may have autism are the repetitive and restrictive behaviors that you will likely notice as unique characteristics of your child. These also can be quite impairing to your child. Most children with ASD require a very strict, rigid routine and sameness in their environments. For example, when the rug in the classroom is changed or moved, or a peer is out sick, the child may have a severe tantrum. Your child might have a tantrum if you drive a different route to school than usual or run an unexpected errand after school. Your child may have hand flapping or be more concerned with the parts of objects: he will just want to spin the wheels on a toy car rather than play with it appropriately. Children with ASD have over-sensitivity and/or under-sensitivity of one or all of their senses. For example, there might be very few foods that they eat due to sensitivities to taste, texture, and smell. They may refuse to brush their hair and teeth or have tantrums when you do these for them. They often refuse to get a haircut. These symptoms make children with ASD appear odd compared to their peers and cause them to be more isolated than they would be if they simply had social impairments (3). Below is a list of red flags regarding these behaviors that may indicate ASD in your child.

Red Flags Related to Unusual Interests and Behaviors
+ Lines up toys or other objects
+ Plays with toys the same way every time
+ Likes parts of objects (e.g., wheels)
+ Is very organized
+ Gets upset by minor changes
+ Has obsessive interests
+ Has to follow certain routines
+ Flaps hands, rocks body, or spins self in circles

By at least the preschool age, you may have concerns over your child's lack of interest in peers, speech delay, "failures in empathy" ("my child does not care if someone is crying or upset"), resistance to change, restricted interests, and/or stereotyped movements. It is common for parents to finally express these concerns to their child's physician or provider, especially when they are worried about their child's inconsistent responsiveness and lack of age-appropriate language, and wonder if their child could be deaf. You may also notice significant problems with your child's transitioning from one task to another without a temper tantrum or handling changes in routine.

Other symptoms are not regarded as core symptoms of ASD but are nonetheless very troublesome and impairing. For example, although tantrums are not a "core symptom" of ASD, you will likely feel that they are the most problematic symptom as they can cause disruption in all environments and make learning and discipline difficult. Undoubtedly, you will note some or all of the symptoms listed below in your child if he or she has ASD (4).

Other Symptoms Common in Those with ASD
+ Hyperactivity (very active)
+ Impulsivity (acting without thinking)
+ Short attention span
+ Aggression
+ Causing self-injury
+ Temper tantrums
+ Unusual eating and sleeping habits
+ Unusual mood or emotional reactions
+ Lack of fear or more fear than expected

These various red flags and sets of symptoms are important for you to know, whether you are starting to notice unusual symptoms in your toddler or whether you have an older child already diagnosed with ASD but are still unsure of what specifically identifies your child as having ASD. Of course, you should not diagnose your child on your own. Please see a professional for an official diagnosis. Sometimes a first-time parent will fail to recognize symptoms or over-recognize symptoms of

ASD. Let the professionals handle the official assessment and diagnosis, but educate yourself on the signs and symptoms. If the signs and symptoms seem to describe your child, then discuss this with your pediatrician immediately. If you still have concern but your pediatrician does not, schedule an appointment with a developmental pediatrician, a child psychologist, or a child psychiatrist.

Once your child has been diagnosed with ASD, there are different ways in which he or she may develop. A small number of children will have marked gains developmentally. Some make slow and steady progress, while others have episodes or waves of improvements intermixed with periods of worsened behavior. Still others may deteriorate and have severe tantrums, self-injury, and aggression. However, in my experience, most children do not get worse, although they may appear to get worse compared to their typically developing peers who do steadily and quickly make progress. Some with ASD seem to plateau in their improvements, while others continue to improve steadily. It has even been noted more recently that some "outgrow" autism. Certainly this is the exception, but I have treated a handful of these very interesting cases. What is clear from the evidence and my experience is that you cannot predict the outcome/prognosis or how quickly things will improve. You cannot accurately predict who will plateau. Predictors of ultimate outcome, based upon some research, are the presence of communicative speech by age 5 and cognitive ability (IQ). However, regardless of your child's current, specific characteristics, there is always hope that he or she will improve, even significantly, over time. Some research even shows improvements into a person's 20s. The earlier your child receives the ASD diagnosis and the earlier therapies are started, the better your child's outcome. There is reason to be hopeful that your child will continue to make strides.

DIAGNOSES THAT MIMIC ASD

As we discussed earlier, there are disorders that can be confused with ASD. These must be ruled out or considered by the professional treating your child before a diagnosis can be made and treatment plans discussed. Neither you, and especially not your clinician, should simply make a diagnosis based on a couple of "red flags" or a few common symptoms. This can easily lead to misdiagnosis. This is why it is very important to be diagnosed by a professional who is adequately trained, competent, and personally comfortable with the routine diagnosis of ASD. A diagnosis of ASD will only be made when full DSM-5 criteria are met. If you are not sure, ask members of the autism community or your child's pediatrician for the name of such a provider in your community. Typically, this is a child psychiatrist, psychologist, or developmental pediatrician.

The most common disorders that can mimic ASD are specific developmental disorders (especially language disorders), sensory impairments (especially deafness), intellectual disability, obsessive-compulsive disorder (OCD), anxiety disorders (especially selective mutism), reactive attachment disorder (RAD), childhood-onset schizophrenia, mood disorders (especially bipolar disorder), and other disorders, since this is not a complete list. In my practice, I have seen ASD misdiagnosed as bipolar disorder many times: some professionals misinterpret autism tantrums as the "rages" of bipolar disorder, as discussed previously.

Language disorders can more easily be mistaken for ASD, especially in the preschooler. These individuals can struggle with language and, as a result, socialization. There are two characteristics that best differentiate children with ASD from those with language disorders: pointing for interest and the use of gestures. If your child can point to things to show you or is able to use other gestures, it is likely there is only a language disorder present.

If your child truly has ASD, he or she would also have repetitive and restricted interests and not only problems with social communication.

RAD can have symptoms similar enough to ASD to make diagnosis more difficult. Children with RAD have difficulties in attachment to caregivers and may respond inappropriately in social situations. For example, children with RAD may fail to attach to their caregivers and act withdrawn or indifferent to their parents. Alternatively, some children with RAD may indiscriminately attach and walk up to a complete stranger and sit in the stranger's lap. The symptoms of RAD can improve with adequate caregiving and therapy.

OCD symptoms can also be seen in those with ASD. However, typically, what the parent thinks of as obsessions are more like circumscribed interests (like my previous example of Dora the Explorer). True obsessions are bothersome to the child, while circumscribed interests or repetitive behaviors associated with ASD are often comforting and even enjoyable. OCD is not associated with significant social or communication impairments like those seen with ASD.

Anxiety disorders may be confused with ASD in some cases. For example, in the anxiety disorder of selective mutism, the child refuses (or is unable) to talk in certain situations or with new people. However, the social and communication problems in those with autism are constant, while they are situational in those with anxiety disorders.

Childhood schizophrenia and ASD can share common symptoms of social impairments and odd patterns of thinking. In ASD, significant hallucinations or delusions are considered to be very rare, but they are common in schizophrenia. And unlike in children with ASD, children with schizophrenia should not have significant communication deficits unless their thoughts are highly disorganized.

COMMON COMORBID DISORDERS

Children with ASD often have comorbid, or co-occurring, disorders. These comorbidities can be as much of a problem as the ASD itself, or even more so. It is important for you to understand the information in this section so that you know that there are disorders or symptoms that your child with ASD might have that can be treated directly. Although there is arguably no medication treatment for the core symptoms of ASD, there are proper and effective treatments for the comorbid disorders in this section that can greatly improve your child's life and functionality.

The most common comorbidities found in children with ASD are ADHD and anxiety disorders. Also, approximately 50% of those with autism meeting full DSM-IV criteria have severe or profound intellectual disability, 35% have mild to moderate intellectual disability, and nearly 20% have IQs in the normal range. However, the older criteria (DSM-IV) for autism were more narrow than for the newer (DSM-5) ASD diagnosis, so the group studied was more severely impaired than a group with broader spectrum ASD. More children with the more recent ASD diagnosis will have higher IQs. Clinical depression (major depressive disorder) is seen in some with ASD, especially in adolescents and apparently in those who have more insight into their symptoms: they may realize how they are viewed by their peers and recognize their deficits. Small studies have noted a possible increased risk of bipolar disorder, tics, and Tourette's syndrome (verbal and motor tics) (1).

Anxieties and phobias can be found in up to half of children with an ASD diagnosis, with many having more than one anxiety and/or phobia. It is very important and helpful to identify these anxieties with your physician so that proper treatment can be provided (with medication or therapy) and potential triggers for behavioral problems can be decreased.

Social anxiety disorder is likely the most common comorbid psychiatric disorder: it is present in about 29.2% of children with ASD. ADHD is a close second, at about 28.2%, and oppositional defiant disorder is third, at 28.1%. Other studies have found higher rates of ADHD (5). In fact, based on my clinical experience, most children with ASD have some degree of impairment from ADHD symptoms such as hyperactivity, impulsivity, and inattention. As such, I often start medication treatment with a stimulant, when appropriate.

Up to two thirds of children with ASD can be considered to also have ADHD, depending on the study. This is because some studies contradict the above 28% figure and suggest a much higher likelihood of ADHD. Regardless of the true risk of ADHD in those with ASD, it is important for you to recognize that ADHD is commonly seen in those with ASD. The identification and effective treatment of ADHD in your child can be quite helpful. It may reduce some of the more significant problems that your child is having in the academic environment and even other social environments. Of those with comorbid ADHD, 84% also have another comorbidity (a third diagnosis) (5).

OCD, according to one study, may be the second most common co-occurring disorder in children with ASD. OCD-like behavior also characterizes many of their early childhood problems, such as insistence on sameness or unwillingness to change routines. Over one third have an obsession or compulsion that limits their ability to interact socially. Many believe that although the OCD is similar in those with ASD, it is not the same; there is a different quality. Sometimes the OCD-like symptoms seen in ASD are not bothersome to the child as they are in those with true OCD. The child with autism may seem to actually enjoy the repetitive behaviors and circumscribed interests, even though these symptoms are impairing from the parent's perspective (3).

Depression can be seen as your child gets older, and especially in adolescence. It may become more common as he or she becomes more aware of the diagnosis or of his or her deficits and the child's differences are less well tolerated by peers. Bullying can be brutal during this period, and those with ASD need to be closely monitored throughout their life for clinical depression. If your child becomes depressed, your healthcare professional may consider medication and/or individual psychotherapy to help. If you feel that your child is depressed, or certainly if he or she mentions suicidal thoughts, get help immediately from a mental health professional. If your child is in imminent danger or with suicidal thoughts with a plan, then present to the nearest emergency department for an evaluation. I would recommend that your child see a psychiatrist regularly regardless so that if any of these symptoms develop, they would be recognized during a regular follow-up appointment.

Disruptive behaviors such as aggression or defiance can also be common. These behaviors can be quite problematic: they can lead to suspensions from school and create difficulties with peers and adults, and with academic participation. This can also cause difficulties for you as the parent, and seeing a therapist to help you with parenting skills (ways to handle your child's behavior better) can be very helpful. At times, medication can be used as appropriate (see Chapter 6), and behavioral therapies can be used as well (see Chapter 8).

Although considered rare, up to 2% of those with ASD may develop schizophrenia compared to just 1% in the general population. If you suspect that your child may suffer from schizophrenia, this should be evaluated by a professional (3).

Some symptoms related to ASD may not always warrant another specific diagnosis but can be problematic nonetheless. Variable behavioral problems can be found in individuals with ASD, including OCD-like symptoms, aggression, self-injury, stereotypies, tics, anxieties, insomnia, and mood symptoms. Children with ASD can have significant mood lability or problems regulating their moods or reactions. They can be over-reactive or under-reactive emotionally and/or physically.

The most common physical abnormalities associated with ASD are epilepsy (with an incidence of 19%) and bowel disorders (12%) (6). Those with ASD frequently have sleep disorders and constipation. You are most likely going to notice that your child will have gastrointestinal problems. Discuss treatments for these medical problems with your child's primary care physician if/when they occur.

Although not a specifically recognized disorder by the American Psychiatric Association, sensory integration disorder or "sensory problems" are common in those with ASD. The DSM-5 now includes these sensory differences as a possible criterion for ASD. Symptoms of these "sensory problems" would be when your child cringes and covers his or her ears at loud noises, refuses to get haircuts or brush his or her teeth, and will wear only certain clothes with specific textures. Another common sign is that your child may become a very picky eater, to the point that he or she eats only two or three different foods. This can be one of a child's biggest problems in some cases.

SCREENING AND DIAGNOSTIC INSTRUMENTS

Screening for ASD should be done for every child during all developmental assessments. This should include questions regarding the core symptoms of ASD at primary care visits and at visits from other providers such as developmental pediatricians, psychologists, psychiatrists, and so forth. Pediatricians are the most likely to see children on a regular basis. As such, pediatricians are on the front lines and carry the heaviest burden of identifying cases of autism. Recognizing this responsibility, the American

Academy of Pediatrics in 2007 recommended that pediatricians screen all 18- to 24-month-old children for ASD (3).

Multiple screening instruments for ASD have been developed. You and/or your child will likely be involved in the use of these screening and diagnostic tools, so it may be helpful for you to be familiar with them in advance. These screenings are often very short and easy to complete. Some are completed by the clinician and others by the parent. A very common screening tool is the M-CHAT (Checklist for Autism in Toddlers). This screens toddlers and is completed by the parent, often during a visit with the pediatrician. It is a simple set of questions. Another screening form that may be used is the CARS (Childhood Autism Rating Scale), which is completed by the clinician (1).

If the screening tool indicates significant symptoms, then a more thorough diagnostic evaluation will most likely be recommended to evaluate more closely for ASD or to finally rule it out. Unfortunately, there is not a biological test such as a lab test, EEG, or imaging study (CT or MRI) that can identify or diagnose an individual with ASD. The diagnosis is strictly clinical and based on a certain number of specific core symptoms of ASD.

A clinical assessment/evaluation of your child is made based upon the information provided by parents and teachers and the clinician's observation and evaluation of the child using the DSM-5 ASD criteria. Typically, this is enough to clearly diagnose your child with ASD. If after this assessment the clinician cannot definitively give your child a diagnosis of ASD but is still concerned regarding possible ASD, a psychological evaluation should be completed by a psychologist well trained in the diagnosis of ASD. Various diagnostic tools are used in these cases, such as the ADOS (Autism Diagnostic Observation Schedule). This involves the clinician rating your child's symptoms with a semi-structured interview. The ADI (Autism Diagnostic Interview—Revised) is another such diagnostic tool.

Your child may or may not need to use these diagnostic tools: the more subtle your child's symptoms, the more likely he or she will need this further testing (1). Hopefully, one day, we will have a test to quickly diagnose ASD early in infancy. This would also make parents feel more comfortable that an accurate diagnosis has been made.

MEDICAL WORKUP OF YOUR CHILD

Every child should have a thorough medical assessment at the time ASD is suspected. This will include a physical exam. This should especially include an evaluation for neurological abnormalities such as increased head circumference, hypotonia (low muscle tone), toe-walking, and so forth (2). A hearing test should also always be done. A Wood's lamp examination should be done for signs of a disorder called tuberous sclerosis, as well as genetic testing. Genetic testing may include a G-banded karyotype, fragile X testing, or a chromosomal microarray. These genetic tests give your physician information that may or may not help in diagnosing your child. I would recommend fragile X testing and the chromosomal microarray. The chromosomal microarray is now the standard of care; medical geneticists and the American Academy of Pediatrics recommend it specifically as the standard of care. This test will ideally give you information on what genetic abnormality caused your child's ASD. However, in my experience, it is difficult to get insurance companies to pay for the chromosomal microarray unless the child is first referred to a geneticist. For this reason, I would recommend seeing a geneticist for genetic counseling. The geneticist will be able to order the genetic testing as well as give you information about the likelihood of having another child with ASD. Most parents want to know this information.

The yield for finding an abnormality on genetic testing is as follows: 2.5% karyotype, 0.57% for fragile X, and 24% for chromosomal microarray. Since there is a higher likelihood that a genetic abnormality will be found with the chromosomal microarray, this is the best genetic test to use if your child has ASD. Any abnormal or indeterminate result from a genetic test requires further testing and genetic counseling. Contrary to what most people may think, low IQ does not predict an abnormality identifiable by genetic testing. Testing specifically for MeCP2 gene may be needed in a few cases to rule out Rett's disorder.

What is not clear is how helpful genetic tests are in treating ASD. If something shows up on the genetic test, there is usually not much that can be done to treat that specific problem at this time. However, this may change in the future (1).

Any other unusual features that you notice in your child, like a history of regression, staring spells, family history of ASD, and unusual facial or other body features, may require additional evaluations by other specialists. Other possible causes of ASD-like symptoms need to be identified or ruled out, such as infections (e.g., encephalitis or meningitis), endocrine problems (e.g., hypothyroidism), metabolic problems (e.g., homocystinuria), trauma (e.g., head injury), toxic exposures (e.g., fetal alcohol syndrome), or genetic problems (e.g., chromosomal abnormalities).

Depending on the results of some of the tests or exams performed, your specialist may suggest that your child undergo an MRI, EEG, or other lab tests (1). Do not be afraid of the tests or the number of tests if your provider believes them to be necessary: it is very important that we correctly diagnose your child. However, it is uncommon for all of the above tests to be needed. Furthermore, it is not important that you know the above in detail, but knowing generally what is involved may provide you with some comfort that your child is receiving a thorough assessment by his or her provider.

OTHER REFERRALS NEEDED

Psychological assessments of your child may be needed not only for diagnosis of ASD (at times) but also for further evaluation of his or her cognitive abilities, deficits, adaptive skills, and other parameters helpful for treatment planning. It may also help the school provide best for your child given his or her IQ, strengths and weaknesses, and learning differences.

Referral to early intervention programs may be suggested even if the clinician is not yet sure if your child is on the autism spectrum, as precious time could otherwise be wasted. Also, if your child is older than 3 and has ASD or even suspected ASD, he or she should be referred immediately to the special education program in the local school district.

All children on the autism spectrum deserve at least an initial assessment with occupational therapy, physical therapy, and speech therapy professionals. Occupational therapy can help with fine motor skills (writing/drawing), balance, imagination, appropriate play, sensory disturbances, and many other important areas of functioning. Speech therapy is essential to any ASD treatment plan and should be started immediately even if ASD is simply suspected; do not wait for an official diagnosis or even a hearing test. Language can be improved significantly with speech therapy and can predict overall outcome and disability. If your child seems to have good language abilities but has ASD, he or she still needs speech therapy to help with the pragmatics of speech. Often children who are quite verbal, as in Asperger's disorder, still have problems with the appropriate use of speech. Also, the meager services that most schools offer for speech and occupational therapy are almost certainly insufficient alone. Please get these therapies outside of the school system as well.

REFERENCES

1. Volkmar F, Siegel M, Woodbury-Smith M, et al. Practice parameter for the assessment and treatment of children and adolescents with autism spectrum disorder. *J Am Acad Child Adolesc Psychiatry.* 2014;53(2):237–257.
2. Huerta M, Bishop SL, Duncan A, Hus V, Lord C. Application of DSM-5 criteria for autism spectrum disorder to three samples of children with DSM-IV diagnoses of pervasive developmental disorders. *Am J Psychiatry.* 2012;169:1056–1064.
3. Harrington JW, Allen K. The clinician's guide to autism. *Pediatr Rev.* 2014;35(2):62–77.
4. Centers for Disease Control and Prevention. Autism spectrum disorder: signs and symptoms. Available at http://wwwnc.cdc.gov/ncbddd/autism/signs.html.
5. Simonoff E, Pickles A, Charman T, Chandler S, Loucas T, Baird G. Psychiatric disorders in children with autism spectrum disorders: prevalence, comorbidity, and associated factors is a population-based sample. *J Am Acad Child Adolesc Psychiatry.* 2008;47(8):921–929.
6. Kohane IS, McMurry A, Weber G, et al. The co-morbidity burden of children and young adults with autism spectrum disorders. *PLoS One.* 2012;7(4):e33224.

4

WHAT CAUSES AUTISM?

The amount of research being done in autism spectrum disorder (ASD) has grown exponentially in recent years, leading to rapidly changing data and statistics. As a result, our understanding of autism is constantly evolving. This makes it difficult for professionals and families to keep up. However, the ever-increasing pace of new developments offers us all hope. There is hope for better understanding of ASD by professionals and for more effective treatments. And there is always hope for a "cure" or at least a plan for the prevention of autism in the generations to come.

The most recent statistics speak to the urgency in solving the autism "puzzle." There have been dramatic rises in autism since at least the late 1980s. Based on the latest available data, which are from the year 2010, the Centers for Disease Control and Prevention (CDC) estimates that 1 in 68 children in the United States has ASD, with the biggest increase in cases being among the higher-functioning patients, African Americans, and

Hispanics. However, based on the data from the year 2000, the prevalence was 1 in 150. This is certainly a frightening jump in prevalence over a 10-year period. Some postulate that this is simply due to better diagnosis, although many studies do not support this. In a previous year, when the data showed that 1 in 88 children had ASD, the CDC noted that ASD was more prevalent than the childhood diseases of AIDS, cancer, and diabetes combined. Typically childhood cancer and diabetes have gotten more attention than autism, at least until recently. But this statistic helps to put the number of children and families affected by autism into perspective (1).

A surprising government survey conducted in 2014 suggests that 1 in 45 U.S. children ages 3 to 17 have been diagnosed with ASD. This is quite a bit higher than the CDC's 1-in-68 figure, but because the new data came from a parent survey, the 1-in-45 figure has not replaced the CDC's number.

I believe the prevalence is truly increasing, but when advocating for children with ASD, I typically state, "Does it really matter whether or not the prevalence is increasing? The rate is still too high." I see ASD overwhelming families and school systems every day. It is already a problem that needs to be addressed regardless of whether the prevalence is increasing. Some people will argue that the incidence of ASD is *not* truly increasing, and they use this as an excuse to do nothing or to dismiss it as not being a "real" problem, attitudes you are likely to experience in the school district and at the state level. There is a serious lack of urgency to put into place the services that our children need. Despite the high numbers of ASD cases given to us by the CDC, these figures still don't capture the full gravity of the situation.

The following are the most recent statistics, based on 2010 data. ASD is five times more common in boys (1 in 42) than in girls (1 in 189). Studies in Europe, Asia, and North America all show similar prevalence rates. Although the averages may be similar globally, South Korea reported a prevalence of 2.6%, which was more than twice the prevalence found in the United States (1%). This may have been due to a better study design that captured all cases and not just a sampling from some U.S. cities as done by the CDC. Regardless, individual cities, counties, and states in the United States have each found different rates (2). Why would these rates differ based on location? What might this tell us about the cause of ASD?

ASD is found to occur in all ethnic groups, races, and socio-economic groups. Autism clearly does not discriminate.

In the United States, it has been estimated that the cost of caring for and treating those with ASD is $35 billion per year. The cost for families per year is $67,000 to $72,000. The lifetime cost internationally is estimated at $4 million per individual with ASD (3). These statistics are important in helping the government understand the need to put more resources into studying ASD, finding more effective treatments, allowing more money to be diverted to the educational system, and providing better long-term care for those with ASD.

POSSIBLE CAUSES OF AUTISM

Although the short answer to the question of what causes autism currently is, "We don't know," we do know that there are multiple different pathways that can result in the phenomenon of autism. This is because there are multiple well-known genetic disorders (see Chapter 3) that are associated with ASD, although the overwhelming majority of cases of ASD still do not have a currently identifiable genetic abnormality.

Children with ASD are often very different from one another, so there is a broad spectrum of what autism "looks like." Many pieces of the puzzle of autism elude us, but we have uncovered some of them. Overall, it appears that ASD is caused by genetic factors, environmental factors, and epigenetic factors (epigenetics refers to how the genes and the environment interact).

In the remainder of this chapter, we will discuss the most recent information regarding the potential causes of autism. As a parent of a child with ASD, I believe this information is important for parents to know. Parents often ask me, "What causes autism?" The information presented here is the latest we have regarding the answer to this question. Knowledge is power. It also provides us with comfort in knowing that scientists are working on uncovering the secrets of autism. And this knowledge offers us hope, and the importance of hope cannot be overstated. Knowing the truth about autism and understanding its likely causes can help remove unnecessary guilt: it challenges parents' initial belief that they "did something wrong" and caused their child to have autism.

BRAIN DIFFERENCES IN ASD

There are some notable brain differences in those with ASD. Electroencephalographic (EEG) abnormalities and seizure disorders are found in as many as 25% of those with ASD. An EEG is the test that is usually used to uncover a possible seizure disorder. This indicates a neurobiological problem.

The fact that such a wide set of symptoms is present in ASD suggests that diverse neural networks (or parts of the brain) are involved. Studies show abnormalities especially in the brain's limbic system, which controls basic emotions such as pleasure, pain, and fear. Functional magnetic resonance imaging (fMRI) has shown difficulties with social and affective judgments as well as problems with facial recognition. Overall brain size increases have been noted in ASD. There are abnormalities in white matter tract development in the brain as well (white matter tracts are involved in communication between brain cells).

The most consistent finding in ASD is the elevation of the neurotransmitter serotonin outside of the brain. Neurotransmitters are the chemicals used by brain cells to communicate with each other. Serotonin is responsible for mood balance. The significance of this elevation is unknown currently. The role of the neurotransmitter dopamine is suggested due to the hyperactivity and stereotyped mannerisms seen with autism and because atypical antipsychotic medications that decrease dopamine levels seem to help reduce some symptoms (4).

GENETIC CAUSES

Parents who have a child with ASD have a 2% to 18% chance of having a second child with ASD. The 18% chance cited is when the newer, broader ASD diagnostic criteria are applied rather than the older, more narrow ones (see Chapter 3). Among identical twins, if one twin has ASD, the other twin has a 36% to 95% chance of also having ASD. In fraternal (non-identical) twins, if one twin has ASD, the other has a 0% to 31% chance of having ASD. Furthermore, ASD is more likely to occur in those with certain genetic disorders. About 10% of children with ASD are found to have fragile X syndrome (1%), tuberous sclerosis (1%), Down syndrome, Rett syndrome (0.5%), neurofibromatosis, or other disorders (2,5,6).

With more recent advances in genetic techniques, researchers have found genetic abnormalities associated with autism on almost every chromosome. Even so, despite the improvements in genetic testing, up to 75% of ASD cases have no measurable genetic abnormality.

Much energy had initially been focused on finding the genetic cause(s) of autism. However, there have not been the expected yields from this research. It seems there is not a simple, single genetic abnormality responsible for the overwhelming majority of autism cases; hence, there is no simple "answer." Also, the "heritability" of autism (the degree to which autism is genetic) was once thought to be much higher (at about 90%), but a recent rigorous study has shown a heritability of only 37%. This would indicate that outside environmental factors and the environment inside the mother's womb are likely more important than the genetic factors. This has led to more focus on the environmental causes of autism in recent years. Another study in the *Journal of the American Medical Association* found a heritability of about 50% when 2 million families were included in the study, but this is still far less than the earlier 90% estimates of heritability. Thus, genetic factors explain at most only half of the risk for autism. The relative recurrence risk of ASD was 10.3 for full siblings, 3.3 for maternal half siblings, 2.9 for paternal half siblings, and 2.0 for cousins. This would mean, for example, that a full sibling (sharing 50% of the genes) has 10 times the risk of autism (7). This information can be used to help families with genetic counseling.

ENVIRONMENTAL CAUSES

Many risk factors for ASD have been uncovered in recent years. For example, parents who have children at an older age (older than 35 for mothers and older than 40 for fathers) have a higher risk of having a child with ASD. Closer spacing of pregnancies also increases the risk. A child who is born prematurely or with a low birth weight has an increased risk of ASD. Also, it is more typical for the first-born child to have ASD. Children conceived in the winter months have a 6% increased risk of ASD (8). Family members of children with ASD have higher rates of learning and language problems and social disability, and possibly increased rates of mood and anxiety disorders.

You may be asking why these are the specific risk factors for ASD, and this is the reason why the symbol for autism is a puzzle piece. We do not yet understand how to make sense of these many puzzle pieces of risk factors to put together the complete puzzle or a clear understanding of autism. For example, does it make sense that the older the parent, the more likely it is that a child will have ASD, even when another risk factor is being a first-born child? In time, I am sure we will understand this.

Vaccines

The issue of childhood vaccinations has been the most controversial theory of autism for lay people and pediatricians alike. The fact that most children are diagnosed with ASD about the same time they are given numerous vaccines has worried many parents. A certain percentage (variable in studies) of ASD cases are regressive (the loss of already acquired developmental milestones) and present around the same time the vaccinations are given. This leaves many parents feeling as if their child was "normal" before the vaccines were given—hence, vaccines are blamed. Initially, the measles-mumps-rubella (MMR) vaccine was linked to autism by a British gastroenterologist named Andrew Wakefield. It was later discovered that his study was full of bias. The journal that published Dr. Wakefield's article retracted the article, but not before setting into motion a great deal of fear and the seemingly unstoppable theory that vaccines cause autism. In more recent studies, the MMR vaccine link with autism has clearly been disproven.

After the MMR link to autism was refuted, the blame shifted to thimerosal (a mercury-containing preservative) in multidose viral vaccines. Even though this too was later disproven as a cause of ASD, to calm the fear of parents, manufacturers removed thimerosal from their vaccines (5). However, the fear of vaccines lives on in the autism community. This causes some parents to refuse to vaccinate their children, leading to other worries for the population as a whole. The internet is full of websites with false information still claiming that ASD is caused by vaccines. This is not true and believing this will make it harder for us to uncover the real cause of autism. Please be careful with anything you read on the internet and discuss your concerns honestly with your doctor.

In response to the concern that some children's immune systems were becoming overwhelmed by receiving too many vaccinations at one time, a 2013 study found no link between the number of vaccines a child was given and the risk for ASD (9). Also, a 2015 study found that the MMR vaccine was not associated with autism even in siblings of children with autism (those at higher risk). These studies should provide much reassurance to parents and the link between vaccines and ASD should be put to rest (10).

Immune Response

Pregnant women who contract a viral or bacterial infection have been found to be more likely to have a child with ASD. It is also believed that the child's ASD may be a consequence of the mother's immune response to the infection and not the infection itself. One study indicated that maternal viral infection in the first trimester and maternal bacterial infection in the second trimester was associated with later ASD diagnosis. There is also evidence that prenatal stress (such as that brought on by an infection) might be more detrimental to male fetuses than female fetuses, leading to the higher incidence of autism in males. However, this does not mean that if you get an infection when you are pregnant, your child will have autism (1).

Premature Birth and Fetal Exposure

Certain exposures have been associated with ASD, such as rubella infection, first-trimester exposure to thalidomide, valproic acid (Depakote; used for seizures or bipolar disorder), terbutaline (used to stop premature labor), and untreated phenylketonuria. One study indicated that prolonged fever during pregnancy was a risk factor (5). According to another recent study, low Apgar scores (a rough measure of the health of the baby at birth) and neonatal conditions needing special follow-up have been identified as risk factors for ASD (11). ASD is also about three times more common in infants born at less than 27 weeks' gestation compared with term infants. Each week of shorter gestation is associated with an increased risk of ASD. Additionally, intracranial hemorrhage (brain bleed) and high-frequency ventilation (newborns on ventilators) are associated with ASD among infants born at less than 34 weeks' gestation (12).

Thus, avoiding infections during pregnancy (as much as is possible) and avoiding the use of medications such as valproic acid, thalidomide, and terbutaline will reduce your child's risk of ASD. You should also get routine prenatal care and follow closely the recommendations of your obstetrician/gynecologist (OBGYN). Good prenatal care can reduce your risk of premature labor and other complications associated with ASD. If you already have a child with ASD, this is still important information as you may want to have another child. You will certainly want to reduce your risk of having a second child with ASD.

Some parents have asked me whether testosterone causes autism. In one study, higher levels of testosterone in the amniotic fluid did increase the likelihood of ASD. However, this could not be the "cause" of ASD because even the individual with the highest testosterone level in the study did not have ASD.

There is growing evidence for a possible "three-hit" hypothesis whereby ASD may result from

1. Genetic predisposition
2. Prenatal stress (infection vs. other)
3. Testosterone surge.

High levels of androgens (testosterone), especially in the male, may increase the vulnerability to prenatal stress in those already more vulnerable genetically. This would also explain the four- to five-fold greater incidence in males developing ASD. But this is only one current hypothesis, and there is not, at this time, anything you can do to reduce testosterone levels in the amniotic fluid—nor would you want to do so at this time (6).

Dietary Deficiencies

There is a hypothesis that ASD, cerebral palsy, and attention-deficit/hyperactivity disorder (ADHD) are all caused by a prenatal insult of some sort followed by an exaggerated inflammatory response in the brain. This prenatal insult may be an infection in the mother or fetus, loss of blood flow to the fetus, an allergy in the mother, or an autoimmune disease (whereby the person's own immune system attacks him or her). This inflammatory response in the fetus may injure susceptible brain cells. A current hypothesis is that this inflammatory response would occur in autism at about 36 weeks' gestation to 2 months after delivery. As the theory goes, our present diets lack enough antioxidants and omega-3 polyunsaturated fatty acids (found generally in vegetables and cold-water fish, respectively) while having too much omega-6 polyunsaturated fatty acids. Omega-6 increases inflammation while omega-3 reduces inflammation. The theory would be that taking omega-3 during the first trimester as well as a powerful antioxidant such as N-acetylcysteine would reduce by 75% the incidence of autism. However, this is only a theory and has not been proven. Taking omega-3 would also not prevent whatever the insult was that caused the problem in the first place (13).

Pediatrics published a case report of a child with autism who improved significantly after vitamin D3 supplementation. It has been proposed that vitamin D plays some role in causing ASD. We know already that vitamin D is important for brain development. Furthermore, lower vitamin D3 concentrations may lead to increased brain size, enlarged ventricles in the brain, and altered brain shape. All of these changes have been observed in those with ASD. For these reasons, children with autism should be assessed for vitamin D deficiency by blood test. However, if your child's vitamin D level is found to be low and your doctor prescribes vitamin D replacement, this does not mean your child's autism will go away. In my practice, it has helped to variable degrees, but it is not a miracle. It should also be noted that even most children without ASD probably have low vitamin D levels. I would ask that your healthcare provider check your child's vitamin D level if it has not already been done. It is something that is easily corrected (14).

Evidence from many fields of medicine has documented multiple medical abnormalities in ASD that are not simply associated with the brain. This suggests that ASD is a whole-body disease or at least of multiple organs. Some such abnormalities deal with inflammation, immune problems, energy generation (mitochondrial systems), the gastrointestinal system, and so forth.

Chemical Exposure

More recently there has been concern over the association of ASD with pesticides, phthalates (found in plastics), perfumes, air pollution, many other chemicals, and electromagnetic fields (8). Experts already know that the environmental toxicants of mercury, lead, arsenic, polychlorinated biphenyls (PCBs), and toluene can cause neurodevelopmental disorders. About 85,000 chemicals have been manufactured in the United States, and of these, 2,800 are used in high volumes with little information existing about their developmental toxicity (15).

Several studies have shown that some with ASD express changes in genes involved in the detoxification (removal from the body) of environmental pollutants. Due to these differences in genes, some people may not be able to remove dangerous chemicals from their bodies as well as others do. These genes have been called "environmental response genes," and more than 100 of these genes may contribute to ASD risk. These genetic differences are thought to increase adverse effects from these environmental toxicants (15).

One review of all recent literature regarding environmental toxicants found that 92% of the 37 studies reported showed an association between ASD and environmental exposures to the following toxicants: pesticides, phthalates, PCBs, solvents, toxic waste sites, heavy metals, and air pollutants. This is concerning, but an association does not mean that these chemicals cause autism (although they may). Most parents are concerned about mercury causing autism, but exposure to methylmercury during pregnancy, such as by mother's eating fish, was not associated with ASD. Childhood exposure to toxicants in the water supply was not associated with ASD. The strongest evidence was found for exposure to pesticides and air pollutants (15).

Heavy Metals

Heavy metal exposure is frequently a concern of parents in my office, but the results are mixed: only 47% of the 40 studies showed higher concentrations of heavy metals in the blood, urine, hair, brain, or teeth of children with ASD. Studies of heavy metals did suggest evidence of a dose–effect relationship: the higher the level of heavy metals in the child's body, the more likely the child was to have ASD. However, this is not conclusive evidence that heavy metals cause ASD or that your child should undergo chelation therapy to remove these heavy metals (see Chapter 7).

Some studies have had limited sample sizes and some bias. We need additional high-quality studies to clarify the relationship between heavy metals and ASD (15).

Pesticides

Pesticides are specifically designed to damage the nervous system of a particular "pest." Thus, it would not be very surprising if they were found to have a significant impact on the brains of unintended targets, including us. The risk of ASD has been found to be increased in children whose mother lived near agricultural applications of organochlorines during the first trimester. More recently, organophosphate insecticides have replaced organochlorines for many residential and agricultural purposes. In 2001, they were banned by the U.S. Environmental Protection Agency in residential products. Higher levels of organophosphate pesticides have been found in the urine samples of pregnant woman who later have children diagnosed with ASD. Also, higher levels of these pesticides in the umbilical cord blood were associated with ASD symptoms in early childhood. Other studies have noted that organophosphates were related to problems with visuospatial performance, memory, motor coordination, and cognitive development, and these are all symptoms similar to ASD (16).

Since the ban on organophosphates for household usage, other pesticides have become more common. Since 2009, over 3,500 products in the United States have been registered that contain synthetic pyrethroids or pyrethrins. Although these have short half-lives (disappear quickly) in humans, pyrethroid metabolites have been found in over 70% of adults. These pesticides are pervasive in our environment and likely unavoidable. Further study of the effects of this chemical on humans and the developing fetus is warranted (16).

Phthalates

Phthalates are chemicals that are used to make plastics more flexible and harder to break. Often called plasticizers, they are used in hundreds of products such as detergents, lubricating oils, vinyl flooring, adhesives, automotive plastics, plastic clothes (raincoats), and personal-care products. These hygiene products are perhaps most concerning as they are more often used by females and nearly unavoidable. These include soaps, shampoos, hairsprays, and nail polishes, and phthalates have been found in 75% of cosmetics as well. Phthalates are also used in plastic packaging film, garden hoses, inflatable toys, medical tubing, and some children's toys. You are exposed to phthalates by eating and drinking foods that have been in contact with products and containers containing phthalates. To a smaller degree, you can be exposed by breathing in air that contains phthalate vapors or dust contaminated with phthalate particles. Young children may have a greater risk of being exposed to phthalate particles because they put their hands in their mouths more often. According to the CDC, the human health effects from exposure to low levels of phthalates are unknown.

The CDC states that certain types of phthalates have affected the reproductive system of laboratory animals. Although no conclusive human study has been conducted, most experts agree that many findings from numerous animal studies may be relevant to humans. Phthalates have been implicated in behavioral problems and possibly ADHD and ASD. Animal studies suggest that phthalates may impact birth outcomes, including gestational age and birth weight, as well as fertility (via lower sperm production). They may even cause anatomical abnormalities related to the male genitalia, at least in animals. Human studies are also evaluating if phthalates may affect the timing of puberty or even cause obesity or asthma.

Phthalates are also associated with changes in body size, conduct disorder, ADHD, and social deficits. The presence of phthalates in the urine of mothers in their third trimester is associated with poorer social responsiveness in the child. A study found that ASD risk was doubled by living in a home that had vinyl (polyvinyl chloride [PVC]) flooring in the children's and parent's bedrooms. PVC flooring is a significant source of airborne phthalates. Both bisphenol A (BPA) and phthalates, in general, are linked to thyroid dysfunction, which could have multiple implications on health as well (16).

BPA is a specific type of phthalate that is a plasticizer found in plastic food wrappings, can liners, plastic drink bottles, baby bottles, and other products. It has estrogen properties. It has been linked to obesity and diabetes. Both obesity and diabetes in the mother have been linked with an increased risk of ASD in her children. Increased BPA levels in mothers were associated with behavioral problems in children. BPA was more recently banned in baby bottles secondary to these concerns. However, it appears that the replacement chemical (BPB) is so similar to BPA that it also is of concern (16).

European governments have restricted the use of phthalates in some cosmetics, baby products, and plastics that typically come into contact with food. In 2009, California prohibited the manufacture, sale, and distribution of products containing more than one-tenth of 1% of any of six phthalates in all childcare products and toys made for children younger than 3 years old. Other states are likely to follow. So far, the United States has not found enough damaging evidence for phthalates and has left it up to manufacturers (17).

As we all know, plastics are everywhere, as are phthalates. Our children eat and drink from plastic containers. The best thing to do as a parent or a pregnant woman is to limit exposure to these chemicals. Here's a list of the most common phthalates, which may come in handy for checking labels:

- DBP (dibutyl phthalate)
- DNOP (di-n-octyl phthalate)
- DiNP (diisononyl phthalate)
- DEP (diethyl phthalate)
- BBzP (benzyl butyl phthalate)
- DEHP (di 2-ethylhexl phthalate)
- DiDP (diisodecyl phthalate)
- DnHP (di-n-hexyl phthalate)
- DMP (dimethyl phthalate)
- DnOP (di-n-octylphthalate)
- BPA (bisphenol A)

What steps can you take to limit the number of phthalates to which you and your family are exposed? Limit the amount of baby care products you use on your baby. Choose products that are phthalate-free. Unfortunately it is not always easy to tell from the list of ingredients, as manufacturers are not required to list phthalates separately, but avoid the above-listed chemicals, which should be mentioned in the ingredient list. Also avoid any product that uses the term "fragrance," as this typically has phthalates in it to hold the scent longer. Even if the product is safe, the container may not be, causing the phthalates to leach from the plastic container to the product. The Campaign for Safe Cosmetics website lists many specific brand-name products and whether they contain phthalates.

Although less convenient, use glass and stainless steel instead of plastic for water bottles, storage containers, baby bottles, and so forth. You will need to use extra caution with glass to prevent breakage. If you must buy plastic bottles, such as for baby bottles or water bottles, look for bottles that are phthalate-free.

New corn-based plastics are now being marketed and are called polylactides (PLA). These are completely biodegradable and considered free of chemical leaching dangers. When buying plastic containers, check the bottom of plastic bottles and choose those labeled #1, 2, 4, or 5. These are generally considered safer. Those labeled #3 may leach phthalates. Plastic labeled #7 may leach BPA and #6 may leach styrene.

Never microwave food in plastic containers and do not put plastic containers in the dishwasher because the high temperatures in the microwave and dishwasher cause the chemicals to leach out of the plastics. As BPA can be leached from the lining of canned goods, choose fresh fruits and vegetables and those in glass containers. Avoid using canned infant formulas; instead, breastfeed or use powdered formula.

Do not buy vinyl (PVC) products, especially if these products may end up in your baby's mouth (products such as teethers, pacifiers, or specific plastic toys). Instead, choose items made from natural products when possible. When you do buy plastics, look for those made of polyethylene or polypropylene plastics rather than vinyl or PVC.

Avoid inhaling phthalates. When painting or using other solvents, be sure the space is well ventilated. Make sure your child is not in the room when you are painting and do not paint when pregnant. Most paints contain DBP (dibutyl phthalate), but you can find natural paints without this ingredient. Also, whenever possible choose non-vinyl shower curtains, raincoats, and lawn furniture. The chemical vapors from these products introduce phthalates into your environment. Clean frequently, as phthalates can end up airborne and in the dust in your home. Wet mopping can help eliminate the chemical. Avoid using air fresheners; even when labeled "phthalate-free," most air fresheners contain phthalates.

Do not become overwhelmed when trying to reduce your exposure, because it is impossible to completely avoid exposure to phthalates or other chemicals. Just do the best you can to reduce your risk.

Pollutants

In one study, mothers who lived near a freeway in the third trimester or at the child's birth were more likely to have children with ASD. This suggests the need to examine more closely the association between air pollutants and autism (18). Other studies have suggested a 1.5 to 2 times increased likelihood of ASD with increased exposure to air pollution. The association of autism and air pollution is greater in males (16).

Electromagnetic Fields

There are known biological effects of extremely low-frequency electromagnetic fields (EMFs) such as from power lines. In 2014, a study showed that mice exposed to EMF had lack of normal sociability, decreased preference for social novelty, and less exploratory activity. However, this has not been studied in humans, and no correlation with ASD has been officially made. Further research is needed to support or refute an association between EMFs and autism (19).

OBGYN RECOMMENDATIONS

To help reduce the risks of ASD and the exposure to chemicals while pregnant, the American College of Obstetricians and Gynecologists (ACOG) has made the following recommendations. Discuss with your doctor all medications that you are taking and their associated risks to you and your child. You should especially discuss risks associated with terbutaline, valproic acid, over-the-counter pain relievers, and psychiatric medications.

ACOG also recommends taking folic acid before and during pregnancy. Research shows that taking folic acid does reduce the risk of autism. Taking folic acid before conception improves outcomes of other neurodevelopmental and behavioral disorders. It reduces the risk of neural tube defects, attention deficits, hyperactivity, and language delay and increases social competence and executive functioning. Taking prenatal vitamins near the time of conception reduces the risk of ASD by 40% (16).

Although cigarettes and alcohol have not been specifically implicated in ASD, they do have multiple known adverse effects on fetal development. Therefore, avoid cigarettes, alcohol, and second-hand smoke.

Eat plenty of fresh fruits and vegetables while pregnant, but wash them thoroughly to remove pesticides. I would recommend buying organic fruits when possible or at least buying organic in those fruits most likely to have high levels of pesticides. I also would recommend organic milk as it would be free of growth hormones and other chemicals.

Eat fewer processed foods. Chemicals from packaged foods (e.g., microwave-ready meals) can leach into the food. These chemicals can include "endocrine-disrupting" chemicals such as BPA and phthalates. As mentioned above, avoid plastics with codes #3, #4, and #7.

Limit or eliminate oily fish and tuna from your diet, especially when pregnant. These oily fish can accumulate DDT (dichlorodiphenyltrichloroethane) and PCBs (polychlorinated biphenyls) in their fat. Tuna can also have high levels of mercury and lead, as can shark, swordfish, king mackerel, and tilefish.

Limit or eliminate use of personal care products (e.g., body wash, perfume) that are strongly scented. These can also contain harmful chemicals. When pregnant and breastfeeding, avoid exposure to strong fumes such as fresh paint, pesticides, fungicides, and solvents, as well as exposure to new furniture, new cars, and non-stick frying pans. This will reduce your exposure to PFCs (perfluorinated compounds).

Perfumes and cosmetics are known to have highly mutagenic, neurotoxic, and neuromodulatory effects. This means that the chemicals in perfumes and cosmetics are known to cause genetic mutations and to harm the brain. The reason these chemicals are allowed into these products is due to a loophole in the Federal Fair Packaging and Labeling Act of 1973, which exempts fragrance producers from disclosing ingredients on labels. Unfortunately, these fragrances are now widely used in other products such as detergents, soaps, cosmetics, food flavorings, and others. Even at very small concentrations, these chemicals have effects on certain cells in the brain called neuroblastoma cells. These chemicals are very likely able to reach the developing fetal brain when pregnant mothers are exposed to these chemicals. Thus, these chemicals have been implicated as a possible environmental cause of ASD and other diseases due to the known ability of these chemicals to mutate genes (2).

According to ACOG, every pregnant woman in the United States is exposed to at least 43 different toxic chemicals. Some health problems associated with exposure to toxic environmental agents are infertility, miscarriage and stillbirth, impaired fetal growth and low birth weight, preterm birth, childhood cancers, birth defects, cognitive/intellectual impairment, and thyroid problems. Pesticide exposure in men is associated with poor semen quality, sterility, and prostate cancer. Pesticides may interfere with puberty, menstruation and ovulation, fertility, and menopause in women. According to ACOG, about 700 new chemicals are introduced into the United States each year, while more than 84,000 chemical substances are currently in use. We do not have safety data on most of these chemicals despite the fact that they are in our air, water, soil, food supply, and everyday products.

CONCLUSION

Many reasons have been proposed for the increasing prevalence of autism. We now know that ASD is not mostly a genetic disease, as once thought. At least half (if not more) of the contributors to ASD stem from environmental factors. There is now legitimate evidence for multiple potential environmental causes. The number of studies trying to uncover the environmental causes of autism has exploded. There are some known genetic abnormalities associated with ASD, but the overwhelming majority of ASD cases (75%) do not have a known genetic cause. The broadening of the definition, better screening, and improved diagnosis are all possible theories for the recent dramatic increase in ASD prevalence. Many studies have explored how much of the increase in ASD is a "real" increase versus simply better diagnosis, and most studies do indicate that there has been a "real" increase. A 2014 study showed that about 75% to 80% of the noted increase in autism since 1988 is due to an "actual increase." Oddly, most of the suspected environmental toxins have either flat or decreasing trends and thus do not correlate well with the corresponding increase in ASD numbers. For example, lead, car emissions, and organochlorine pesticides have decreasing trends over recent years. But there are still plenty of harmful chemicals in our environment (23). Many more high-quality studies are needed to clarify the environmental and genetic causes of ASD. Although you will not be able to avoid all chemical exposures, there are many things you can do to decrease this exposure and thereby reduce your child's risk of ASD.

REFERENCES

1. Tchaconas A, Adesman A. Autism spectrum disorders: a pediatric overview and update. *Curr Opin Pediatr.* 2013;25:130–143.
2. Centers for Disease Control and Prevention. Key findings: trends in the prevalence of developmental disabilities in U.S., 1997–2008. http://wwwnc.cdc.gov/ncbddd/develpmentaldisabilities/features/birthdefects-dd-keyfindings. Published 5/19/2011. Accessed Dec 2015.
3. Reichow B, Barton EE, Boyd BA, Hume K. Early intensive behavioral intervention (EIBI) for young children with autism spectrum disorders (ASD). *Cochrane Database Syst Rev.* 2012;10:CD009260.
4. Volkmar F, Siegel M, Woodbury-Smith M, et al. Practice parameter for the assessment and treatment of children and adolescents with autism spectrum disorder. *J Am Acad Child Adolescent Psychiatry.* 2014;53(2):237–257.
5. Harrington JW, Allen K. The clinician's guide to autism. *Pediatr Rev.* 2014;35(2):62–77.
6. Schaafsma SM, Pfaff DW. Etiologies underlying sex differences in autism spectrum disorders. *Frontiers Neuroendocrinol.* 2014;35:255–271.
7. Sandin S, Lichtenstein P, Kuja-Halkola R, Larsson H, Hultman CM, Reichenberg A. The familial risk of autism. *JAMA.* 2014;311(17):1170–1777.
8. Zebro O, Iosif AM, Delwiche L, Walker C, Hertz-Picciotto I. Month of conception and risk of autism. *Epidemiology.* 2011;22(4):469–475.
9. DeStefano F, Price CS, Weintraub ES. Increasing exposure to antibody-stimulating proteins and polysaccharides in vaccines is not associated with risk of autism. *J Pediatr.* 2013;163(2):561–567.
10. Jain A, Marshall J, Buikema A, Bancroft T, Kelly JP, Newschaffer CJ. Autism occurrence by MMR vaccine status among US children with older siblings with and without autism. *JAMA.* 2015;313(15):1534–1540.
11. Polo-Kantola P, Lampi KM, Hinkka-Yli-Salomaki S, Gissler M, Brown AS, Sourander A. Obstetric risk factors and autism spectrum disorders in Finland. *J Pediatr.* 2014;164(2):358–365.
12. Kuzniewicz MW, Wi S, Qian Y, Walsh EM, Armstrong MA, Croen LA. Prevalence and neonatal factors associated with autism spectrum disorders in preterm infants. *J Pediatr.* 2014;164(1):20–25.

13. Strickland AD. Prevention of cerebral palsy, autism spectrum disorder, and attention deficit-hyperactivity disorder. *Med Hypotheses.* 2014;82(5):522–528.

14. Jia F, Wang B, Shan L, Xu Z, Staal WG, Du L. Core symptoms of autism improved after vitamin D supplementation. *Pediatrics.* 2015;135(1):e196–198,

15. DA Rossignol, SJ Genuis, RE Frye. Environmental toxicants and autism spectrum disorders: a systematic review. *Transl Psychiatry.* 2014;4:1–23.

16. Lyall K, Schmidt RJ, Hertz-Picciotto I. Maternal lifestyle and environmental risk factors for autism spectrum disorders. *Int J Epidemiol.* 2014;43(2):443–464.

17. De Cock M, Maas YG, van de Bor M. Does perinatal exposure to endocrine disruptors induce autism spectrum and attention deficit hyperactivity disorders? *Acta Paediatr.* 2012;101(8):811–818.

18. Volk HE, Hertz-Picciotto I, Delwiche L, Lurmann F, McConnell R. Residential proximity to freeways and autism in the CHARGE study. *Environ Health Perspect.* 2011;119(6):873–877.

19. Alsaeed I, Al-Somali F, Sakhnini L, et al. Autism-relevant social abnormalities in mice exposed perinatally to extreme low frequency electromagnetic fields. *Int J Devel Neurosci.* 2014;37:58–64.

20. Bagasra O, Golkar M, Rice LN, Pace DG. Role of perfumes in pathogenesis of autism. *Med Hypotheses.* 2013;80(6):795–803.

21. Nevison CD. A comparison of temporal trends in united states autism prevalence to trends in suspected environmental factors. *Environ Health.* 2014;13:73.

22. Connolly JJ, Hakonarson H. Etiology of autism spectrum disorder: a genomics perspective. *Current Psychiatry Rep.* 2014;16:501–509.

23. Anagnostou E, Zwaigenbaum L, Szatmari P, et al. Autism spectrum disorder: advances in evidence-based practice. *Can Med Assoc J.* 2014;186(7):509–519.

AUTISM'S EFFECT ON
THE WHOLE FAMILY

The impairments associated with autism spectrum disorder (ASD) not only affect the individual with ASD, but also dramatically impact the parents, caregivers, family, teachers, school system, peers, and the community in general. The overall responsibility is great and felt by everyone who comes into contact with the individual with ASD. In this chapter, we will focus on ASD's effect on the family. First, we will discuss what is known about how ASD typically impacts the whole family. Second, we will discuss how this family impact causes a reciprocal negative effect on the child with ASD, which may then diminish positive outcomes of interventions. Lastly, we will discuss the extent to which parental involvement is needed during treatments or interventions. I will show how certain interventions may reduce stress and the negative effects on the family and the child with ASD.

It is my intention and hope that a discussion of what is "normal" in families affected by ASD will provide you with a greater understanding of ASD and the recognition that you are not alone in dealing with these challenges. This should lessen your sense of isolation and allow you to feel that your family dynamic is less "odd" and unique than you likely currently feel. As knowledge is power, some of the latest evidence and research will be shared. Being armed with this information will provide you with the confidence to tackle the typical difficulties associated with autism. You will learn how to be more resilient and avoid the most common pitfalls.

IMPACT OF ASD ON THE FAMILY

The symptoms of ASD present a unique set of challenges for parents and the family as a whole. Thus, it is not surprising that research in this area indicates that caregivers of those with ASD have decreased parenting efficacy, or a reduced belief in their own parenting skills. These caregivers also have more parenting stress and increased mental and physical health problems. This is true even in comparison to the caregivers of children with other developmental disorders. On average, parents experience additional stressors like financial strain, more time pressures, higher divorce rates, and lower levels of family well-being. These additional stressors not only affect the caregiver but may, in turn, negatively affect the person with ASD and reduce improvements from interventions. Furthermore, when the child improves via a particular intervention, the extra time and expense related to the intervention may further stress the parent. Therefore, the way ASD affects the family must always be considered when interventions are pursued.

Our understanding of ASD is continuously changing, and even its cause remains unclear (see Chapter 4). The most effective and most appropriate treatment regimen is not well established or wholly agreed upon. Many providers or professionals (primary care physicians, psychiatrists, neurologists, psychologists, teachers, etc.) are not well trained in caring for or treating individuals with ASD. Furthermore, most health insurance companies do not cover even the most evidence-based treatments, not to mention that most treatments are not covered at all or sometimes not enough. This makes it difficult or even impossible to get the treatment your child needs and arguably deserves. These dilemmas may leave you feeling alone to navigate the problems involved in caring for your loved one. This may add to the hopelessness, isolation, and grief that you already experience. Even the most educated caregiver, including myself, struggles to get appropriate care for his or her child. There is no real road map yet, and there are many snags along the way. From personal experience, I can tell you that it feels like a constant struggle, with many people and institutions (e.g., school system, insurance company, Medicaid, disability) to battle.

Interestingly, caring for a child with ASD has significant negative effects on the parent and family regardless of the severity of autism or the time that has passed since the initial diagnosis. In fact, caregiver stress typically occurs long before the actual diagnosis. Some parents note differences in development as early as 6 months, but most report specific concerns around 18 months, well before the average age of diagnosis at 4 years old according to the Centers for Disease Control and Prevention (CDC). Some research even indicates an older average age of first diagnosis (6–7 years old), especially in those with the diagnosis previously known as Asperger syndrome. The period of time between the parent's concern that something is "not right" and the time of diagnosis is very stressful. Any delay in diagnosis only increases your anxiety and worry.

In my experience, professionally and personally, the suspicion of ASD is typically first noted by parents, family members, and/or speech therapists rather than by primary care physicians, psychologists, or psychiatrists. This likely affects how and when the announcement of autism is made. The "bad news" may be delivered by someone who is poorly equipped to handle the telling of this news or who cannot direct the family properly toward the first steps that need to be taken. This may leave you, as the parent, feeling lost and more distressed than you otherwise would be had you been told and educated by the most appropriate professional. In fact, in one study, approximately 63% of parents expressed dissatisfaction in the way that the ASD diagnosis was announced.

While hearing the diagnosis of "autism spectrum disorder" for your child is painful, most often parents also express relief that they now have an explanation for their child's difficulties and a better way of understanding their child.

PARENTING EFFICACY (AM I A GOOD PARENT?)

One of the impacts of ASD on the parent is by way of parental self-efficacy: parents' own belief regarding their ability to parent their child. With typically developing children, parents with high parental efficacy tend to show more effective parenting in the face of challenging behaviors. On the other hand, parents of children with disabilities typically have low parental efficacy, which has been associated with increased parenting stress.

Caregivers of children with ASD may be unique in having lower parenting self-efficacy for a few reasons. First, the definition and understanding of autism and the treatment are continuously changing. This leaves parents unsure of how to get their child help, and causes them to question the most appropriate way to parent their child. Second, the typical delay in diagnosis also means that the parents have often not been using the best parenting strategies for their child for long periods of time, thus causing them to doubt their parenting ability. Lastly, parents feel ineffective at parenting because their child's problems in social communication cause the parents to not understand the child's wants or needs. They may not feel able to meet their child's emotional or physical needs, causing anger, frustration, guilt, or a range of other emotions.

A couple of studies have shown that brief parent management training or parent-focused interventions can increase parental self-efficacy. Parents report fewer behavioral problems in their child after these interventions, meaning that these interventions likely have a direct impact on the child (1). This is why one of the first referrals for the family of a child with ASD is for parent training and/or for Applied Behavioral Analysis (ABA) therapy (see Chapter 8), which typically includes parent training as well.

According to research, parents' knowledge after the ASD diagnosis continues to grow over time. While overall the gain in knowledge regarding ASD is helpful, the source of much of this knowledge appears to be the internet. Unfortunately, these sources may not have been validated by professionals. This information may not be accurate and can lead parents to pursue inappropriate or even dangerous therapies. These internet searches may add to parents' overall confusion regarding the best interventions or treatments, or even regarding the diagnosis. Please use caution when doing research via the internet, and discuss important questions or issues with your provider.

PARENTING STRESS

Another way that ASD affects you, as the parent, is through "parenting stress." Parenting stress is the stress and tension revolving around the task of parenting. Parents of children with ASD have higher levels of parenting stress than those of children who are typically developing or those with other types of developmental delay or special healthcare needs. The factors that contribute to parental stress in caregivers of children with ASD include the child's cognitive impairment, behavioral problems, internalized distress, mood disturbances, functional dependence, hyperactivity, lack of self-care abilities, noncompliance, low adaptive functioning, language deficits, learning disability, imposed limits on family opportunities, need for care across the lifespan, toileting difficulties, sexual expression, social difficulties, and the high likelihood of remaining in the home.

Interestingly, research has shown that the level of cognitive impairment does not seem to change the level of parenting stress. Also, those with a "high-functioning" (higher IQ, more verbal, etc.) child with ASD do not have less parenting stress. Furthermore, neither the level of language/communication deficits nor the severity of stereotypies (stemming) changes the level of parenting stress. Thus, it appears that it is the unique combination of the pervasive behavioral, emotional, and functional problems, not the core symptoms of ASD, that creates and exacerbates parenting stress. Furthermore, parenting stress is associated with more negative parent–child interactions, harsh authoritarian parenting, child behavior problems, and ineffective implementation of interventions.

Studies have shown that parents raising children with ASD have significantly more stress than those parents raising children with Down syndrome, fragile X, cerebral palsy, or specific learning disorders. This suggests that it is the child's behavioral problems that add the most stress. Studies indicate that the attention-deficit/hyperactivity disorder (ADHD) symptoms of inattention, hyperactivity, and impulsivity induce stress in parents, as do the deficits seen specifically in ASD, such as problems with social communication and odd ritualistic and rigid behaviors. Often those with ASD also have ADHD. Children with ASD who also have significant tantrums, aggression, and self-injurious behavior are likely to increase parents' stress levels even more (2).

There are numerous ways in which ASD affects mothers and fathers differently. Mothers of children with ASD appear to have more parenting stress than fathers. Also, as children get older, mothers appear to have less stress, while fathers' stress is consistent throughout childhood. Researchers suggest that possibly "acceptance" of ASD deficits is related to lower stress in mothers as children get older. According to research, the emotional dysregulation (irritability/moodiness) of the child increases maternal stress, while behavioral problems impact fathers most. Maternal stress is affected not only by the child's behavior or difficulties but also by the father's mental health. However, the mental health of the mother does not directly affect the stress of the father. Mothers also show higher levels of parental involvement compared to fathers, which might explain the higher stress in mothers. The father's primary coping strategy seems to come from his work outside of the home, while the mother's comes from social support (3). Understanding these mother/father differences may help you understand where your child's other parent is coming from and that he or she may be experiencing things differently.

There are several risk factors for increased levels of parenting stress, which is often impacted by the coping strategies used and by the extent of social support. Not surprisingly, the more isolated the family is, the higher the parental stress level. Furthermore, if the parent has delayed or given up "life plans" as a result of the child with ASD, parental stress is greater.

As a parent, you must reduce your stress level as much as possible. Getting more social support, learning better coping strategies, and taking some time for yourself will help you to manage your stress better. Have your child stay overnight with his or her grandparents or a family friend you trust. Hire a babysitter who understands autism and go out at least once a month.

Do not let inappropriate anxiety that your child will not be taken care of or that he or she will be a burden for the sitter inhibit a well-deserved and needed break.

Parents, especially mothers, experience more stress when parenting their children with ASD than when parenting the unaffected siblings. Surprisingly, findings indicate that parents raising children with ASD are not simply stressed in general, since their stress is reported as normal when parenting the unaffected siblings. Both mothers and fathers have more depressive symptoms when raising a child with ASD, even compared to parents of children with ADHD (2).

It appears that parents with ASD or ADHD have more difficulty parenting their children or less ability to cope with the behavioral problems of their children. Hence, they report more stress and more depressive symptoms. It is intriguing that it is primarily mothers with ADHD and fathers with ASD who have increased parenting stress. This is likely due to typical parenting roles. For example, mothers are more likely to be involved in organizing the household, making sure children get to school on time, and other activities that require effective time management and organizational skills. A mother with ADHD would struggle more with these duties. Fathers are typically more involved with recreational and educational activities. A father with ASD would struggle more with the social communication needed to effectively manage these duties. Thus, if you are a parent who has ASD or ADHD yourself, you should seek treatment as well. It will make your life and your family's lives much easier and less overwhelming.

EFFECT OF ASD ON PARENTS' HEALTH

ASD has also been shown to affect parents' mental and physical health with a general decrease in parental well-being. In comparison to parents of typically developing children, parents of children with ASD have an increase in mental health problems, especially depression and anxiety. One small study showed that 33% of mothers and 17% of fathers were clinically depressed. In the same study, 6% had clinically significant anxiety. In another study, almost 30% of parents experienced moderate to severe levels of anxiety, while nearly 20% were clinically depressed. Furthermore, about 80% of the parents felt sometimes "stretched beyond their limits" (1). This certainly is a feeling with which most of us can identify. Dealing with the child's behavioral problems contributes most to the depression and anxiety. These statistics remain significant even in educated mothers without significant socioeconomic burden.

Mothers of children with ASD experience greater anxiety, depression, and overall distress than do fathers. Also, mothers are more affected than fathers by the health of their child and spouse. Single mothers have more distress than those who are married, even when socioeconomic factors are taken into account. This suggests that having a partner or at least another caregiver is at least somewhat protective against maternal depression. Interestingly, lower socioeconomic status did not by itself increase parental stress. However, higher parental self-efficacy and family support contributed most to better parent mental health (1).

Parents of children with ASD also have greater physical health problems than do parents of typically developing children. They experience higher levels of fatigue as well. The sleep quality of both the father and of the child predicts a mother's depressive symptoms. It is not clear by what mechanism parents would have more health problems except that the higher levels of stress intuitively would take their toll over time. Please attend regular check-ups with your primary care physician. Do not be embarrassed to discuss the stress you are under in caring for a child with ASD. You should discuss this with your primary care physician as well as seek mental health treatment when appropriate. Take care of your physical and mental health needs. Mental health treatment may include seeing a counselor, psychologist, or psychiatrist, or even attending a support group. You, your child, and your family need you to remain in good physical health and be around for a long time. Your child needs you to be healthy now and in the future.

The best way to reduce your stress as a parent is to develop a solid support system with family and friends, both to confide in as well as for respite. You will need breaks from the stress or "me time." You can then return to your child refreshed and with a better perspective. You need to recognize your limits and use coping skills to deal with stress, anxiety, and depression. Lean on your spouse or significant other and work as a team. If you are a single parent, utilize whatever family or friends you have for emotional support and for babysitting. When things get too difficult to handle, such as if severe depression or severe anxiety develops, seek help from mental health professionals.

Amazingly, despite the worsened mental and physical health of parents of children with ASD, they appear to have overall better relationship closeness with their children than parents of typically developing children. It has been proposed that the diagnosis of the child itself may protect the parent–child relationship. Parents tend to view the child as less responsible for his or her behavior even though they are upset about the behavior. They are not as likely to be "angry" with the child; they are more likely to "blame" the child's behavior on the ASD and not on the child. Also, parenting practices impact the parent–child relationship. For example, mindful parenting practices, defined as "clear, calm mind that is focused on the present moment," have been shown to "decrease aggressive behavior, noncompliance, and self-injury in children with ASD and are also associated with increased maternal satisfaction with parenting skills and child interaction" (1).

HARDSHIPS OF PARENTING A CHILD
WITH ASD

Approximately 85% of individuals with ASD have significant impairments in cognitive abilities and/or adaptive living skills that limit their ability to live independently. This means that it is likely that parents or other family members will have to provide some amount of assistance for the duration of the individual's life. This may then negatively color caregivers' perception of their own future, as this lifelong responsibility carries with it a host of difficulties. In one study, 50% of parents aged 50 or older with children with developmental disabilities still had their children living with them versus only 19% of those with typically developing children (1).

One third to one half of children with ASD also have additional problems or disorders that impair everyday functioning. Some of these symptoms include inattention, hyperactivity, anxiety, and depression. Also, up to 40% to 60% of children and adolescents with ASD have an intellectual disability. These other associated problems are shown to increase parenting stress more than the core symptoms of ASD or the child's level of intellectual functioning (4).

It is likely that the degree of impact that behavioral problems have on parents is related to what the parents attribute as the cause of the behavior and how much control they believe the child has over his or her own behavior. Likely due to the fact that mothers on average spend twice as much time with their child with ASD as do fathers, they are more likely to feel that the behavioral problems are more influenced by environmental triggers and that the child has more control over his or her behavior (4).

Interventions that change parental attributions of the behavioral problems in the child with ASD would likely reduce parenting burden and stress. Ideally, the focus of such an intervention would be emphasizing to parents that both the child and the parent have more control over the behavioral problems than they believe. Furthermore, there are therapies to help with these problem behaviors that do give both parent and child more control over these behaviors. One example is Applied Behavioral Analysis (ABA) therapy (see Chapter 8). The other fact to illuminate in such an intervention is that behaviors are not constant or stable over time, and they are not always simply related to the ASD or inherent child traits. This is typically also worked on in ABA therapy as external triggers are often identified. This provides relief and instills hope in the family dealing with very frustrating and challenging behaviors (4).

There are some interesting facts regarding ASD and family dynamics. On average, mothers report a closer relationship with the child with ASD over the child's lifespan as compared with fathers. Fathers' report of the closeness of the parent–child relationship depends upon the age of the child and the amount of time spent with the child. Fathers should take heart in the fact that the older the child, especially from adolescence to adulthood, the closer is the relationship. Also, the less time the child spends in the home, the closer is the relationship with the father (4),

HOW THE ENVIRONMENT AFFECTS THE CHILD WITH ASD

Environmental or psychosocial factors also impact children with ASD. These factors influence the degree of additional psychological problems experienced. Family poverty is associated with greater emotional and conduct problems (stealing, skipping school, destruction of property, etc.). Also, household chaos is a risk factor for conduct problems. Unfortunately, maternal warmth, involvement of the caregiver, and home organization do not relieve the effect of poverty on overall increased psychological problems. However, a mother's emotional warmth is associated with fewer conduct problems and lower levels of hyperactivity. Thus, family poverty, low maternal warmth, and household chaos are risk factors for significant behavioral problems in children with ASD. We cannot always do much to change our family's financial situation, but we can all show more warmth to our children. It may be that maternal warmth could be a key target for intervention to reduce worse behavioral outcomes in children with ASD. For this reason, it is advisable to express warmth to your child. Sometimes with all of the stress, we forget to do this.

ASD'S IMPACT ON THE MARRIAGE

Children with ASD have an impact not only on the parents themselves but also on the marital relationship. Parenting stress, child behavioral problems, and marital conflict engendered by the burden of autism may contribute to a higher divorce rate. In one study, the divorce rate was twice as high as in families of typically developing children. This risk also extended into the child's early adulthood, as children with ASD have been found to be negatively affected by parent conflict, despite lower overall social awareness of the marital strife. Parents who stay married are still noted to have lower marital satisfaction, which impacts the entire family. It also affects the reported parenting experience of the individual parents, especially in fathers, and appears to negatively impact the sibling relationships of children with ASD (1).

Low marital satisfaction and high stress are typically associated with divorce. Both of these factors are present on average in families with a child with ASD. Despite this, parents may choose to stay together to ensure that they can provide better for their child, especially financially. Families may also remain together because "it is safer to live in discord than to face the unknown change that marital separation inevitably brings" (5). As one mother jokingly stated about her husband, "Oh, he is not going to miss even a minute of this fun" in reference to the stress of their daily lives. She indicated that they would not be getting divorced no matter how unhappy they were, and they would essentially be living together forever to raise their child.

The most important point for you to understand is that raising a child with ASD brings with it many unique stressors that are likely to affect your family and your marriage negatively. Thus, you need to be careful to fortify your marriage as much as possible. Spend time together as a couple. I suggest a date night at least every other week. Try not to argue about the petty things because you have much more important considerations. Be kind to your spouse. After all, you better than anyone else know how difficult your lives are and that you both deserve some slack. If you find your marriage floundering, seek marital counseling.

ASD'S IMPACT ON SIBLINGS

Although there is little research about siblings of children with ASD, some things are clear. It will come as a relief to many that most typically developing siblings report positive relationships with their siblings with ASD. It has generally been understood that siblings must deal with unusual pressures such as potentially receiving less parental attention and time than their sibling with ASD, dealing with poorer communication and social reciprocity from their sibling, and often being embarrassed by their sibling's different and difficult behavior. However, it is thought that siblings may benefit from being a teacher and social helper of their sibling with ASD. I have noted this to be most often the case, both in my own family and among my patients' siblings. As always, however, there are exceptions. Some of these exceptions may be related to the unaffected sibling's personality or his or her own mental health problems.

Unfortunately, according to one study, sibling closeness may lessen over time. More often positive relationships are reported when the sibling with ASD is younger. Interestingly, however, parents are less positive about the sibling relationship than the unaffected sibling themselves. Parents are found also to overestimate the unaffected sibling's understanding of the impact of ASD on the whole family. Perhaps, as has been suggested, this leads to siblings blaming themselves for family difficulties (1). It is commonly known in my profession that we should pay special attention to the siblings of children with ASD because they have unusual stressors and likely feel more responsibility than they should. Please make sure, as the parent, to notice significant anxiety, depression, behavioral problems, and other important symptoms in these siblings. Ideally, in your community there should be a support group for the siblings of children with ASD.

THE COST OF ASD

Families also have practical considerations that become part of the economic burden of ASD. There are numerous financial difficulties. Often, one parent is unable to work because of the stressful environment and many demands associated with ASD. There are frequent time pressures, including the provision of more support and accommodations for the child's education. There is a greater investment of time and money in healthcare and therapies. Likely most difficult is the increased need for vigilant parenting, as much more supervision is needed. Additionally, there is the never-ending need for advocacy for the child in every area, including with family, doctors, therapies, insurance companies, and most definitely the educational system.

The economic cost of ASD for the family is staggering. The financial cost of raising a child with ASD is at least three times greater than the cost of raising a typical child (3). It has been estimated that it costs $3 to $5 million dollars more to raise a child with ASD than it does to raise a typical child. The cost increases more for a child with severe cognitive impairment. This financial burden is even more concerning given that a study has found that treatment outcomes are significantly predicted by socioeconomic status (1).

A 2014 study explored the financial impact of ASD on the family by comparing financial and employment issues relative to the disorders of ASD, ASD plus intellectual disability (ID), ID only, and fragile X syndrome. Financial burden was experienced by 60% of families with children with fragile X, 52% of those with a child with ASD plus ID, 39% of those with a child with ASD only (without ID), and 29% of those with a child with ID only (without ASD). The percentages of parents who quit employment because of the child's condition were 40% of those with a child with fragile X, 46% of those with a child with ASD plus ID, 25% of those with ASD only, and 25% for ID only (6).

These statistics prove what you already know very well: it is very difficult to work and have a child with ASD, especially if you are the primary caregiver. Over time, parents may need to "trade off" who acts as the primary caregiver. For example, if the child is aggressive, the father may need to take over more control as the child gets older and bigger.

Families living in states with higher per capita spending for children with disabilities report less financial burden. According to one study, 78% of families with children with ASD had healthcare expenditures for their child in the last 12 months. Forty-two percent reported expenditures over $500 and 34% reported spending more than 3% of their income on these expenditures.

However, I would argue that had the study included what *should* be spent by the family on appropriate and evidence-based treatments and therapies, these numbers would easily be higher (7).

Families living in states that enacted legislation mandating autism services coverage were 28% less likely to report spending more than $500 for their children's health costs. This provides support for advocates' arguments that this legislation will reduce caregivers' financial burdens. Such legislation is currently being contemplated in some states and has already been enacted in many. However, the coverage is often minimal or has significantly low age limits. Most advocates will tell you that while the legislation does not go far enough, "it is at least a place to start" (8).

Mothers of adolescents with ASD were found to spend more time on housework and childcare and less time on leisure activities than mothers of typically developing children. On average, mothers of children with ASD work 8 fewer weeks per year outside of the home than mothers of children with other mental health problems. These factors lead to more stress and more financial burden, which then likely also impacts the child with ASD (1).

QUALITY OF LIFE AND WELL-BEING

Families of children with ASD are found to have higher overall negative quality-of-life effects than those of children with ADHD or typical children. For mothers, quality of life depends upon the relative burden they take on compared to fathers. For fathers, quality of life depends upon their own absolute burden (1).

One study showed that the subjective well-being of caregivers of children with ASD was significantly lower than that of the general population. The low level of subjective well-being in the areas of "future security" and "leisure activities" points to the difficult home life. This shows that parents are quite worried about the child's future, especially given the lack of resources in securing the child's future. There is much uncertainty and fear regarding their future. There is little to no time for leisure activities due to behavioral issues and the demands of caring for the individual with ASD (9).

Social support has been found to decrease parental stress and adverse physical health outcomes. Also, those who find positive meaning in caregiving have a higher subjective well-being. Making peace with the diagnosis, overall acceptance, and finding meaning likely contribute to positive health and good coping styles.

Thus, social support, self-esteem, and positive meaning in caregiving decrease the effect of stigma on the subjective well-being of the caregiver. Ideally, interventions can be made to increase these positive, protective factors. Stigma can be reduced by community programs aimed at reducing stereotypes and improving education about ASD. Also, outreach programs and insurance companies should recognize the benefits of respite care in the lives of the families and individuals with ASD.

WHAT SHOULD I DO?

As a caregiver you should work on increasing your own self-esteem and seek more social support. Leisure time and respite care must be a larger priority for you. You should seek mental health treatment if you begin to feel depressed or experience anxiety or other problems. Consider individual psychotherapy and use medications if/when needed (but only under a doctor's supervision). Do not be afraid to ask for help. Getting help for yourself will positively impact your child as well, so do it for your child even if you do not want to do it for yourself. You are the most important resource in your child's life. If you are not functioning well, it WILL affect your child.

COPING AND ACCEPTANCE

Parents of children with ASD often use various positive coping strategies such as information seeking, support from family and friends, use of community resources, and methods of stress management. Unfortunately, parents also have been known to use poor coping strategies such as self-blame.

Generally speaking, there are five positive coping skills that increase the likelihood of positive moods: Problem Focused, Social Support, Positive Reframing, Emotional Regulation, and Compromise Coping. Distraction and Emotional Regulation can often result in improving negative moods. Many of these positive coping strategies can be learned in family or individual therapy.

There are four styles of coping that are often associated with less positive moods: Escape, Blaming, Withdrawal, and Helplessness. Problem Focused, Blaming, Worrying, and Withdrawal coping styles are also associated with worsened negative moods.

Perhaps intuitively, many parents can make sense of or meaning out of their difficult parenting experiences. This increases their ability to cope and is often related to religious, spiritual (see Chapter 11), and cultural issues.

One recent study of parents of children with ASD found that psychological acceptance decreased the effect that the child's behavioral problems had on parenting stress or parents' well-being. The effects of acceptance decreased paternal depression as well as maternal anxiety, depression, and stress.

You should move toward acceptance and search for meaning in order to cope more effectively. Seek support from family, friends, and the religious community.

SOCIAL SUPPORT

Daily social support has been shown to predict the daily moods of parents of children with ASD and is associated with less overall distress, better mood, less depression, increased parenting efficacy, and decreased parenting stress. Support from within your family often results in levels of "optimism" being increased. Support from family and support from friends were associated with more positive well-being of the mother. Unfortunately, chronic parenting stress is correlated with the parent's perception of having less social support. This may mean that these parents may not always realize how much support they have, and they may not utilize it as much as would be possible based on these faulty perceptions.

Other parental characteristics are known to decrease support. Single parents have been found to have less social support. This includes divorced parents. This likely adds to the already significant difficulties experienced by divorced families.

Problems with social support seem to be common in families of children with ASD. Social withdrawal is sometimes used as a coping style, but this is maladaptive and leads to less social support. This then has an enormous negative impact on the parent and even the child with ASD over time as they become more isolated. Stigma also causes isolation. Parents may lose friends or have a hard time getting support from parents of typically developing children. Hence, it is logical that two thirds of parents have reported being part of an autism support group. You too should rely on an autism support group to facilitate more social support for you and your family.

There appear to be five main areas with which parents of children with ASD struggle: dealing with challenging behavior, lack of support, dealing with judgments from others, impact on family coping, and the importance of appropriate support. The challenging behaviors that are noted to be most problematic are tantrums, repetitive behaviors, and aggressive behavior. Tantrums are felt to be often unpredictable and difficult to manage, often happening when there are changes in routine or environmental changes in general. Parents also worry about their child being excluded from peers or bullied because of these behaviors.

Many parents find that the most difficult part of the child's tantrums or behavioral problems is the perceived judgment by others. Parents typically feel that other parents judge their parenting or even may think that the child is simply "naughty." Parents feel guilt or shame in public with their child. This has also been the most difficult part for me as a parent of a child with ASD. I often wanted to "lose my cool" and yell out that I was a child psychiatrist and that my child had autism. I wanted to say, "I'm not a bad parent and my child is not a bad child. She was just having an autism tantrum." However, after a while you become very humble and not easily embarrassed. You learn to accept it and not worry about the perceptions of others. It takes a while to reach that point, but I do believe most of us get there. I have also realized that it is not a "bad thing" to get to this point. It is part of acceptance. It is the acceptance of my own child for who she is, of other people's inappropriate reactions, and of my own feelings of anger in challenging public situations.

Support is hard to come by for parents of children with ASD. Most of us experience a sense of exhaustion and feel that we get little to no break. It is difficult to find a babysitter, even from within your own extended family, because of the child's behavioral problems. Some parents describe grandparents as helpful for short periods of time, while others describe them as not understanding ASD or judging them as "bad parents." Most parents also describe getting little help from external organizations. Parents also worry very much about who will help support their child when they are no longer living.

Although parents love their children with ASD, the impact on the family is immense. Parents describe "never-ending" stress, referring to the chronicity of the behaviors and issues unique to ASD. Other parents state, "It consumes you" or "It is a nightmare." I have seen parents with symptoms resembling those of posttraumatic stress disorder, apparently as a result of frequent and persistent stress and tantrums. Many parents feel despair and certainly initial or prolonged grief. Parents often experience a decrease in their self-esteem and often feel they are failures at parenting. Parents also can feel rejected if their child refuses to interact with them. Siblings also may be jealous of the time that parents spend with the child with ASD. Siblings have reported to me that they wished they had autism too so that they would get more attention. Also, siblings can be embarrassed by the behaviors of the child with ASD.

Support from other parents of children with ASD can be helpful. There is a sense that they will not judge you and that they can understand. Also, ideas and strategies for dealing with behaviors can be shared. This reduces isolation. Furthermore, community resources that are difficult to come by can be shared. By talking with other parents, caregivers can often focus on the positive attributes of their own child. For example, if someone else's child has never spoken, you may feel very grateful that yours can speak. The recognition that "it's not as bad as it could be" is a sort of coping strategy. It is important to "count your blessings." You should try very hard to focus on the positives. Of course, it can take years to get to this point.

Parents generally describe schools as unsupportive and lacking the experience and expertise needed. I have personally and professionally found school systems to be woefully inadequate and at times purposely inept due to "lack of resources." Fortunately, there are some amazing teachers who very much care about our children and do their best with the resources given to help our children achieve their potentials more fully. Although you will likely be naïve at first regarding the school system, as was I, be cautious and informed. In my opinion, there is a clear conflict of interest: the more resources they give to your child, the more money they lose. The number of individual education plans (IEPs) or IEP money given to the school district has been frozen many years ago. Thus, they do not have much interest in giving IEPs even when they are clearly needed. Once your child has an IEP, make sure it is followed as written. The already meager resources are likely to be depleted as the number of children diagnosed with ASD grows (see Chapter 9) (3).

Very often parents feel like "shut-ins," unable to leave home as they fear taking their child with ASD out in public. This reduces potential leisure time for the parent and child. It also increases isolation and adds to the feeling of leading a very "not normal" life.

The way in which the family adapts, copes, and functions impacts the child with ASD. It is not simply a matter of the child with ASD affecting the rest of the family; the relationship is clearly bidirectional. Parenting stress has been shown to lessen the positive effects of therapeutic interventions. Of note, the more spending on respite care for parents, the less often the child is hospitalized. However, increased spending on child therapies was not shown to reduce hospitalizations. This would seem to imply that the better the parental well-being, the fewer behavioral problems the child is likely to have. It has been shown clearly that higher parenting stress leads to higher behavioral problems in the child with ASD. Depressed mothers are also less engaged with their children, and decreased parental responsiveness is associated with delays in language development and in joint attention (1).

Families of children with ASD are also less likely to engage in community activities, and this further decreases quality of life for the child with ASD as well as lessening social learning opportunities. Families are less likely to attend religious services or participate in organized activities, and children are more likely to miss school. For those of us with children on the autism spectrum, this is obvious. Our children often have tantrums and at times embarrass us or their other family members, causing us to retreat from these activities. They train us to avoid these situations. These activities typically are just a hassle and not enjoyable. We get tired of the stares or the unsolicited parenting advice. Often even the child is uninterested. However, continue to try to engage in these activities in order to make progress for your family and for your child with ASD.

INTERVENTIONS/THERAPIES

There are a wide variety of interventions/therapies for ASD. In one study, an average of seven different interventions were used in a child with ASD. Within the autism spectrum there is also much variability in individual symptoms in both type and severity. Research into the efficacy of individual treatments is limited and debated. Also, there are not studies to indicate what interventions may be best for the specific child given his or her unique set of symptoms or problem areas. Thus, parents are left to determine for themselves, with little help or education, which treatment is best for their child (1).

During most ASD interventions, parents are directly or indirectly involved, especially during early interventions. Caregiver participation in these interventions is necessary. Parent involvement in therapies provides many benefits, such as better insight into the child and generalization of therapies at home and in everyday life, leading to improvements in the parent–child, marital, and sibling relationships (1).

Interventions can help parents gain a better understanding of what their own responsibilities are in helping their child. They may also give parents the support and confidence they need. Unfortunately, due to high levels of anxiety, parents can be so overprotective that the intervention's effects are diminished and the child cannot make progress, especially with independent skills.

We will discuss behavioral interventions and other non-medication treatments in Chapter 8. For now, please understand that participation in and understanding of your child's therapies will improve the outcomes of these therapies. In helping your child, knowledge and participation are very important.

Understanding the effect of ASD on sibling relationships, your marriage, your physical and mental health, and the physical and mental health of your child's other parent is very important in order to avoid common mistakes and to provide some comfort in knowing that what you are experiencing in an "abnormal" situation is "normal." Recognizing how to strengthen yourself and your family to reduce stress and other problems is a must. Seek out social support, respite care, and interventions for yourself and your family. Do not be afraid or ashamed to ask for help.

REFERENCES

1. Karst JS, Van Hecke AV. Parent and family impact of autism spectrum disorders: a review and proposed model for intervention evaluation. *Clin Child Fam Psychol Rev.* 2012;15:247–277.
2. van Steijn DJ, Oerlemans AM, van Aken MAG, Buitelaar JK, Rommelse NNJ. The reciprocal relationship of ASD, ADHD, depressive symptoms and stress in parents of children with ASD and/or ADHD. *J Autism Dev Disord.* 2014;44:1064–1076.

3. Ludlow A, Skelly C, Rohleder P. Challenges faced by parents of children diagnosed with autism spectrum disorder. *J Health Psychol.* 2011;17(5):702–711.

4. Hartley SL, Schaidle EM, Burnson CF. Parental attributions for the behavior problems of children and adolescents with autism spectrum disorders. *J Dev Behav Pediatr.* 2013;34(9):651–660.

5. Freedman BH, Kalb LG, Zablotsky B, Stuart EA. Relationship status among parents of children with autism spectrum disorders: a population-based study. *J Autism Dev Disord.* 2012;42:539–548.

6. Ouyang L, Grosse SD, Riley C, et al. A comparison of family financial and employment impacts of fragile X syndrome, autism spectrum disorder, and intellectual disability. *Res Dev Disabil.* 2014;35(7):1518–1527.

7. Parish SL, Thomas KC, Rose R, Kilany M, Shattuck PT. State Medicaid spending and financial burden of families raising children with autism. *Intellect Dev Disabil.* 2012;50(6):441–451.

8. Parish S, Thomas K, Rose R, Kilany M, McConville R. State insurance parity legislation for autism services and family financial burden. *Intellect Dev Disabil.* 2012;50(3):190–198.

9. Werner S, Shulman C. Subjective well-being among family caregivers of individuals with developmental disabilities: the role of affiliate stigma and psychosocial moderating variables. *Res Dev Disabil.* 2013;34:4103–4114.

10. Midouhas E, Yogaratnam A, Flouri E, Charman T. Psychopathology trajectories of children with autism spectrum disorder: the role of family poverty and parenting. *J Am Acad Child Adolesc Psychiatry.* 2013;52(10):1057–1065.

11. Hartley SL, Barker ET, Seltzer MM, et al. The relative risk and timing of divorce in families of children with an autism spectrum disorder. *J Fam Psychol.* 2010;24(4):449–457.

12. Jones L, Hastings RP, Totsika V, Keane L, Rhule N. Child behavior problems and parental well-being in families with autism: the mediating role of mindfulness and acceptance. *Am J Intellect Dev Disabil.* 2014;119(2):171–185.

PSYCHOPHARMACOLOGY: SHOULD
I USE MEDICATIONS FOR MY CHILD?

There are numerous ways that a child might first present to a child psychiatrist. Most patients who present to my office are referred by pediatricians or therapists because the parent or the professional suspects that the child has autism spectrum disorder (ASD). Sometimes, parents bypass the primary care physician and present directly to whomever it is that they perceive to be the expert on ASD: this could be a developmental pediatrician, child psychiatrist, child psychologist, or child neurologist. Other times, they present their child to me as a "last resort" because they do not know what else to do and are reluctantly considering medications. These parents may have been in denial, avoiding diagnosis altogether, or their child may have already been diagnosed with ASD and they have been avoiding a discussion of medications.

The first question I expect that most parents would ask is, "Can medications cure autism?" However, most parents seem to already understand that the answer to this is, "No." Although medications cannot cure ASD or even technically treat the "core symptoms" of autism, they often do treat some of the most problematic and impairing symptoms associated with ASD. For example, to the parent who is desperate for relief from severe tantrums ("meltdowns"), aggression, irritability, and/or self-harm behavior, an atypical (second-generation) antipsychotic medication can seem like a miracle despite the fact that it is not curing the underlying autism. Although we will discuss atypical antipsychotics in detail further in this chapter, briefly they are a class of medications approved by the U.S. Food and Drug Administration (FDA) that help to treat tantrums, aggression, and other symptoms associated with ASD.

A multitude of impairing symptoms and comorbid disorders are associated with ASD, and many of these symptoms can be treated with medications. I will mention studies throughout this chapter so that it is clear that I am not speaking only from my personal and professional experience but also from real data. It is also helpful to have some information from studies so that you know what is typical to expect from children with autism and from medications. For example, one study of 487 schoolchildren with ASD used a survey of teacher and parents and found high rates of the following problems: easy frustration (60%), inattention (50%), hyperactivity (40%), tantrums (30%), irritability (20%), anxiety/fearfulness (13%), self-harm (11%), destruction of property (11%), and physical fighting (5%). Some studies have also found the presence of intellectual disability to be about 50% and the likelihood of a comorbid disorder, in general, to be 80%. The most common comorbid (co-occurring) disorders have typically been found to be social anxiety disorder, attention-deficit/hyperactivity disorder (ADHD), and oppositional defiant disorder. One study found the following comorbidity rates: specific phobia, 44% (most commonly fear of needles or crowds); obsessive-compulsive disorder (OCD), 37%; ADHD,

31%; separation anxiety disorder, 12%; and major depressive disorder (clinical depression), 10%. Other studies have found much
higher rates of ADHD. However, the point here is that a child
with ASD is likely to have other treatable diagnoses or problems
that can impact his or her functioning. There are symptoms and
disorders that we can treat despite the current lack of an autism
"cure" (1).

Your doctor might recommend one or more of a variety
of medications to help your child with symptoms or disorders
associated with ASD. These medications are referred to as psychotropic medications (medications used for mental health and
behavior) and are frequently used to treat disorders or problems
associated with ASD. Recent studies have shown that about 27%
to 40% of youth with ASD have received psychotropic medication
(2). A 2013 study of over 33,000 children with ASD found that
64% had filled a prescription for at least one psychotropic medication. In this same study, 35% were taking two or more psychotropic medications, while 15% were taking three or more. Thus, it is
not at all unusual for children with ASD to be placed on psychotropic medications. The types of medications used and the symptoms that they treat are the subject of this entire chapter. This
chapter is meant to educate you on what medications are available
for specific symptoms that your child may experience now or in
the future. My intention is to make you feel more comfortable
with the use of medications if they are appropriate for your child's
unique set of symptoms. Use this chapter as a resource and as a
reference. Discuss these medications and your child's symptoms
with your doctor (3).

Studies have shown that increasing age, the presence of
comorbid disorders (ADHD, depression, anxiety, OCD, etc.),
greater intellectual disability, and Asperger's syndrome (as
opposed to autism) are all factors that make psychotropic medication use more likely. (As mentioned in Chapter 3, the previous

diagnoses of autism and Asperger's syndrome, among others, have been collapsed into ASD.) If your child has these characteristics, it may be more likely that he or she will need medication. The global market for ASD treatments is extensive, estimated at $2.2 to 3.5 billion. Also, children with ASD have medication costs that are eight to nine times greater compared to children without ASD. Discuss the situation with your healthcare provider or a social worker if you have difficulty paying for your child's medication. Pharmaceutical companies also have patient assistance programs for patients having difficulty affording their medications, and many times these family income brackets are fairly generous (1).

The use of medication can help your child to function better in his or her environment and to further benefit from and participate in therapies and educational services. For example, if your child is too aggressive and irritable to participate in educational activities, then it will be nearly impossible for him or her to achieve full potential, academically and socially. Reducing aggression and irritability with an atypical antipsychotic, for example, will intuitively lead to a wide range of improvements that otherwise would be impossible. Thus, your child can now participate more fully in educational activities, speech therapy, socialization, Applied Behavior Analysis (ABA) therapy, family activities, and much more. This allows your child to make more progress over time. Also, research indicates that there is a crucial window of opportunity when your child's brain is most malleable. The younger the child, the more malleable is the brain. The more therapies the young child receives, the better the outcome and later functioning. For example, studies have shown that if a child receives two years of ABA therapy before the age of 7, there are significantly greater gains than if this therapy is initiated at a later age. This is not to say that therapy at any age is not helpful, but I provide the above information to explain the reason that early intervention is necessary in terms of therapies, educational interventions, and even medications when appropriate.

In practice, the first thing that you as the parent may say to me is that you are hesitant to use medications because "I have heard about all of the bad side effects" or "I do not want my child to be a zombie." Many of your concerns may be based on inaccurate information (from the internet, commercials, lawyer ads, etc.) and the stereotypes and stigmas perceived to be associated with psychiatric treatment. Adding to this fear and stigma, your child may have previously seen a psychiatrist or a primary care physician who had misdiagnosed your child or who lacked adequate training or expertise to effectively treat him or her. This often places a layer of mistrust between me and you that takes quite a while to overcome. So let's talk about the medications available and what to expect so that you can be informed when you speak with your doctor. Keep in mind that you should have a thorough discussion of risks, benefits, alternatives, side effects, and warnings. At all times, your doctor will be weighing the benefits and risks of each medication to decide whether or not the benefits outweigh any risks.

What follows in this chapter is a significant but coherent discussion and education about the medications most commonly used to treat the most problematic symptoms and comorbidities related to ASD. My hope is that you will be more educated regarding these medications if they are recommended to you and more comfortable in using these medications should they be appropriate for your child. I do not want you to wait to use medications (if appropriate) simply due to fear, mistrust, or misinformation. Also, my own child is on or has been on many of these medications as well: I would not recommend or discuss medication that I would not consider for my own child.

WHAT SYMPTOMS CAN BE TREATED WITH MEDICATIONS?

The most common symptoms associated with ASD that can be treated are those of ADHD, irritability, aggression, self-harm behavior, OCD or OCD-like behaviors, insomnia, and the common comorbidities of depression and anxiety. This is not an exhaustive list of ASD-associated symptoms or comorbidities that can be treated, but certainly these are the most common. The medications most likely to be used to treat ADHD are stimulants and non-stimulant ADHD medications. Atypical antipsychotics are the medications most commonly used to treat significant irritability, aggression, agitation, and/or self-harm behavior often associated with ASD. Selective serotonin reuptake inhibitors (SSRIs) are the medications most likely used to treat depression, multiple types of anxiety, OCD, potentially insistence on sameness, and repetitive behaviors. Also, multiple medications are used to treat the common problem of insomnia. These will be discussed in the following sections.

STIMULANTS

It has been estimated that between 13% and 85% of children with ASD also have ADHD. In my experience, the overwhelming majority of patients who have ASD also have ADHD. If your child has some level of difficulty and impairment with the symptoms of inattention, hyperactivity, and impulsivity, he or she may be diagnosed with ADHD. These symptoms can be significantly impairing and troublesome at home, at school, and in other social settings. Sometimes treating these ADHD symptoms alone can bring significant relief for your child and your family. The use of stimulants in those with ASD is on the rise, with a five-fold increase from 2003 to 2010. I believe that this statistic is often used to show how stimulants are being over-prescribed, but I would argue the opposite: it is just as likely that physicians are catching on to the fact that most children with ASD also have impairing ADHD symptoms (4).

Stimulant medications in children with ADHD, but without ASD, have a response rate of 70% to 80%. Thus, these are very effective medications for the majority of children with ADHD and they typically have few, if any, significant side effects. However, research has shown that these medications are less effective and cause more side effects on average in children who also have ASD. In those with both ADHD and ASD, the response rate is closer to 50%. The most common side effect in those with ASD is irritability. The most worrisome possible side effect is increased aggression or agitation. For this reason, the "start low and go slow" approach is recommended when starting stimulants in children with ADHD and ASD. This means that you and your physician should start at a lower-than-typical starting dose of a stimulant and increase the dose slowly to avoid or decrease the likelihood of these potential side effects. It is really important that you follow the doctor's instructions carefully about how much medication to give. Children with ASD often cannot communicate that they are having side effects such as abdominal pain, nausea, headache, and so forth. You, as the parent, should recognize that any worsening of behavior or mood could indicate a physical or mental side effect (1,5).

A common question that you may have about any medication and especially stimulants is, "How do I get my child to take the medication?" This can be difficult, especially if the child is unable to swallow pills. Problems with swallowing pills or even taking liquid medications are common in many young children but more so in children with ASD as they typically have sensory aversions to many textures, tastes, and smells. However, stimulants come in various forms, such as pills that must be swallowed, capsules that can be opened and sprinkled on food or dissolved in water, liquids, chewables, and patches that can be applied to the skin. Even though it sounds impressive that so many forms of stimulants are available, it can still be difficult to get children on the autism spectrum to ingest a medication if they can feel the sprinkles on their tongue (in the food) or taste the medication even when dissolved or in liquid form. Also, the patches can cause irritation to the skin, or your child may take the patch off secondary to a sensory aversion.

Since it is likely that most children on the autism spectrum have ADHD and because stimulants take effect on the first day they are given, I often start with a stimulant trial after assessment for ADHD. The most common exception is when I see a child with severe aggression and tantrums. In this case, an atypical antipsychotic may need to be started first so that the stimulant medication does not worsen the child's aggression or tantrums. Although you should always follow your doctor's recommendations, I believe this is important information that you should know because it can save time in getting your child better more quickly.

Although all of the FDA-approved ADHD medications are typically used to treat those with ADHD and ASD, methylphenidate is the only stimulant that has undergone significant research and has showed efficacy in those with autism. Methylphenidate comes in a variety of forms. Amphetamine/dextroamphetamine mixed salts (Adderall or Adderall XR) may be prescribed, but in my experience this specific stimulant typically causes more side effects than other stimulants in children with and without ASD, mostly in terms of mood lability (mood swings), irritability, and potentially aggression. However, I have had cases where Adderall XR works better and with fewer side effects than methylphenidate. This is not common, however. There is clear evidence for using methylphenidate in those with ASD and ADHD, but there are no randomized, double-blind, placebo-controlled trials of Adderall in this population (2).

Methylphenidate is a psychostimulant medication that is moderately effective in treating ADHD in children with ASD. It is particularly effective for hyperactivity as it works on chemicals or neurotransmitters in the brain called norepinephrine and dopamine (3). Common trade names that this medication is known by are Ritalin, Ritalin LA, Ritalin SR, Methylin, Methylin ER, Concerta, Metadate, Metadate CD, Quillivant XR, Quillichew ER, Daytrana, Aptensio XR, and others. Also, there are many generics offered for methylphenidate products. Although the above formulations all contain the same chemical compound, each is released differently into the patient's system such that one of these compounds may be more effective or better tolerated (causing fewer side effects) than another. I have quite often seen this in my patients, especially with differing responses and/or side effects between immediate-release and extended-release forms. So if your child fails to respond to a trial of one form of methylphenidate, your doctor may give a trial of another form of methylphenidate.

The largest double-blind, placebo-controlled trial (a high-quality trial) was conducted in 72 children with ASD and ADHD, ages 5 to 14. The response rate was 49%, specifically for hyperactivity. Remember that hyperactivity is not simply "bouncing off the wall": it includes excessive talking, being fidgety, not waiting one's turn, being unable to stay seated, and so forth. Reducing this symptom could help your child make remarkable progress in his or her education and even socialization. It is hard to participate effectively in therapies, education, friendships, and family activities when you cannot sit still (4,5).

In this study, 18% of patients discontinued the medication due to adverse effects such as irritability. Thus, irritability needs to be monitored by you and your child's physician, especially to see if the benefits of the medication outweigh this potential increase in irritability. In other studies, preschool children (ages 3–5) with ADHD and ASD showed a 50% response rate, but half of the children experienced adverse effects. Preschool-age children are more likely to have side effects than older children, and with less effectiveness. In general, side effects are mild, but in some cases the adverse effects on behavior and mood may not be worth the benefits gained in reducing inattention, impulsivity, and hyperactivity (4). Clinically, when a child with ASD and ADHD is taking a stimulant medication, improvements are typically noted not only in hyperactivity but also in inattention and impulsivity. Sometimes, in my experience, improvements are also observed in socialization (to a small degree), communication, aggression, irritability, frustration tolerance, and "moodiness." One of the odd things about methylphenidate is that it can decrease irritability and aggression in some people while increasing these symptoms in others (4,5).

Dosing of methylphenidate may vary quite a bit, depending on the individual child. Table 6.1 provides information about stimulant dosing and duration of action. Some children need relatively low doses, while others need higher doses. If your child needs a higher dose, this does not necessarily mean that your child has "worse" ADHD. The need for a higher dose is more closely related to your child's metabolism of the medication or your child's individual genetics. Side effects, if present at all, may fade within a couple of days to a couple of weeks. If the side effects are severe, such as frequent and uncontrollable crying or agitation and aggression, then call your doctor immediately. The medication may need to be stopped and another medication considered. The most common side effects of the stimulants are decreased appetite, headache, abdominal pain, weight loss (especially in the first month), more difficulty falling asleep, and increased irritability. If irritability is worsened, it may be when the medication is in

Table 6.1. ADHD Medications

Class	Drug Name	Form	Duration
Amphetamine Stimulants	**Adderall** (dextroamphetamine/amphetamine)	Short-acting	4–6 hours
	Dexedrine (dextroamphetamine)	Short-acting	4–6 hours
	Dextroamphetamine extended release	Long-acting	6–8 hours
	Adderall XR (dextro-amphetamine/ampheta-mine extended release)	Long-acting	8–12 hours
	Vyvanse (lisdexamfetamine)	Long-acting	10–12 hours
Methylphenidate Stimulants	**Focalin** (dexmethylphenidate)	Short-acting	4–6 hours
	Methylin (methylphenidate)	Short-acting	3–4 hours
	Ritalin (methylphenidate)	Short-acting	3–4 hours
	Metadate ER (methylphenidate extended release)	Intermediate-acting	6–8 hours
	Methylin ER (methylphenidate extended release)	Intermediate-acting	6–8 hours
	Ritalin SR (methylphenidate sustained release)	Intermediate-acting	4–8 hours
	Metadate CD (methylphenidate extended release)	Intermediate-acting	8–10 hours

(*continued*)

Table 6.1. Continued

Class	Drug Name	Form	Duration
	Ritalin LA (methylphenidate extended release)	Intermediate-acting	8–10 hours
	Concerta (methylphenidate extended release)	Long-acting	10–12 hours
	Quillivant XR (methylphenidate extended release)	Long-acting	12 hours
	Focalin XR (Dexmethylphenidate extended release)	Long-acting	6–10 hours
	Daytrana patch (methylphenidate)	Long-acting	10–12 hour
Nonstimulants *Selective norepinephrine reuptake inhibitor*	**Strattera** (atomoxetine)	Long-acting	24 hours
Alpha-2 agonist	**Intuniv** (guanfacine extended release)	Long-acting	24 hours
	Guanfacine	Short-acting	6–8 hours
	Clonidine	Short-acting	4–6 hours (tablet)
	Catapres	Long-acting	24 hours (patch)
	Kapvay (clonidine extended release)	Long-acting	24 hours if tablets given twice daily

Table 6.1. Continued

Class	Drug Name	Form	Duration
Antidepressants (off-label use for ADHD)	**Wellbutrin** (bupropion)	Short-acting	4–5 hours
	Wellbutrin SR (bupropion sustained release)	Long-acting	12 hours
	Wellbutrin XL (bupropion extended release)	Long-acting	24 hours

the child's system or as the medication wears off, typically in the midafternoon if the medication is an extended-release stimulant.

The biggest concern in the recent past has been the potential of stimulants to induce an arrhythmia (irregular heartbeat). Your doctor may recommend that your child get an electrocardiogram (EKG) before starting to take a stimulant. If there is a family history of sudden death or your child has any known heart malformations or heart murmurs, your doctor will likely recommend an EKG in consultation with a cardiologist before your child can receive a stimulant medication. Although this may concern you as a parent, these medications have a proven record of being very safe and effective. Ask your doctor if you have further concern about this, especially for your child's specific situation. At every visit with your doctor, vital signs (including heart rate and blood pressure) and weight should be obtained. This is to monitor for the rare cases of stimulants increasing blood pressure or heart rate, decreasing weight, and preventing steady growth.

All stimulants last for differing lengths of time, depending on the medication type (Adderall vs. Ritalin), whether it is an extended-release or immediate-release form, and which form it comes in (patch, capsule, sprinkles, etc.). Ask your doctor or pharmacist how long the medication is expected to last so you can note and predict benefits and side effects and correlate them with the medication start time as well as its wearing off. For example, if the medication is helping but is wearing off too soon, your doctor may add an immediate-release medication in the afternoon when the extended-release stimulant wears off to decrease ADHD symptoms for longer during the day. However, the drawback to this additional afternoon dose is that appetite can be reduced longer and it may take longer for your child to fall asleep at night. Alternatively, the doctor may decide to change your child's medication to a different extended-release stimulant that will last longer throughout the day.

I prefer to start with Concerta or another form of long-acting methylphenidate for the treatment of ADHD associated with ASD. I have found, in my clinical experience, that this medication causes fewer side effects than the other stimulants, on average, in this population. I realize that you do not have a say for sure on which stimulant is given first, but some physicians with less experience with ASD may not have a preference for which stimulant is chosen first. In this case, you could ask to use a particular one first or at least ask your doctor why he or she is choosing a particular stimulant first. Unfortunately, your health insurance coverage may also dictate which medication is tried first.

My second preferred stimulant to use in those with ASD is Vyvanse in terms of efficacy and rate of side effects. Thus, if a patient has a poor response or side effects with a trial of long-acting methylphenidate, I will typically give a trial of Vyvanse. This strategy is also advisable because this would mean trying a stimulant in a different family of stimulants as the second choice. Adderall (amphetamine salts) and Vyvanse are most similar to each other and can be thought of as being in the same stimulant family. The other stimulant family would include methylphenidate (Ritalin, Concerta, etc.) and dexmethylphenidate (Focalin,

Focalin XR). It is advisable to try the opposite stimulant family if one stimulant in the family has failed. However, even stimulants within this same rough family can act quite differently in the individual. For this reason, I am rarely opposed to giving all four different stimulants a try before giving up on stimulants for the treatment of ADHD. I would recommend that you not give up on stimulants because of one "bad" medicine trial. Of course, it's up to you and your doctor to decide on the specific medications tried and the order of medications.

If your child is having troublesome side effects but the medication is doing a good job treating the ADHD symptoms, your doctor may suggest that another medication be used to help treat the side effect. For example, if your child is having more difficulty falling asleep and has had significant weight loss and poor appetite, your doctor may prescribe a medication such as mirtazapine (Remeron) that can be used to increase appetite and help with sleep. It is given once daily, at night. Another option is cyproheptadine (Periactin), which may also be used to help as an appetite stimulant without significant sedation. It is given twice daily, 30 to 60 minutes before meals.

If your child is having significant side effects and not much benefit with a specific stimulant, then it is still likely that a different stimulant medication will provide significant benefit and without significant side effects. Be sure to share all signs and symptoms with your doctor so that he or she can consider a different stimulant. Do not give up. Sometimes the first medication is not the best one for your child. I have seen parents struggle with trying four different stimulants before finding the right one for their child. Typically, it is the first medication that works well, but sometimes it takes a couple of trials. You have to be persistent. I am grateful for the families who are willing to trust me and allow a couple of different trials when needed. They never regret it. The best feature of stimulants is that they work the first day that they are tried, unlike most other medications in psychiatry, which can take weeks or months to produce the full therapeutic effect. Thus, a brief trial of a couple of days is often all that is needed. Also, if your child has a "bad reaction" to the medication such as worsened irritability, don't worry. It will usually last for only a few hours.

If you have tried a couple of stimulants and the side effects were too significant and/or the effect was too small, you and your doctor may want to consider adding or changing to a nonstimulant.

NONSTIMULANTS

The nonstimulants can be used as a first-line medication for ADHD treatment. However, because overall they are less effective than stimulants at decreasing ADHD symptoms, they are generally used after stimulant trials have failed. Nonstimulants can be used alone to treat ADHD or together along with a stimulant. Nonstimulants take longer than stimulants to produce noticeable benefits. It takes 2 to 4 weeks to show full therapeutic effects, so you will have to be patient. Also, these benefits can be less dramatic. Nonstimulant medications include guanfacine, guanfacine ER (Intuniv), clonidine, clonidine ER (Kapvay), and atomoxetine (Strattera).

Nonstimulants are often used when the maximum dose of a stimulant for the child's weight is being given but is not helping enough to control ADHD symptoms. In this case, a nonstimulant can be used along with a stimulant so they can work synergistically to decrease ADHD symptoms. If the side effects from a stimulant do not allow the maximum dose to be used, giving the nonstimulant along with the stimulant may minimize the overall total dose of stimulant needed. This, in turn, decreases the side effects from stimulants such as decreased appetite, weight loss, abdominal pain, insomnia, and irritability.

One of the first nonstimulants used was clonidine, which was initially used for treating high blood pressure. We now know that it has many other uses. Clonidine is modestly effective in treating irritability and hyperactivity in children with ASD. It is used to treat the overall symptoms of ADHD, especially hyperactivity and impulsivity, but it is less likely to be as helpful with focus as stimulants are (4,5).

Clonidine is available as a patch or a pill. It can be sedating and, thus, has been found to be helpful for the treatment of insomnia. For this reason, it is often used by child psychiatrists and pediatricians as a sleep aid, especially in children with ADHD and/or ASD. For insomnia, it is typically given at night only. We will discuss treatments for insomnia at greater length in a later section of this chapter. The most common side effects of clonidine are drowsiness, sedation, and decreased activity. It is because of its possible sedative effect that clonidine is not as commonly used to treat ADHD symptoms. To treat ADHD symptoms significantly with this medication, it would need to be given three or four times per day. Some children are too sedated with this dosing. Also, having your child take a medication this often is very difficult. Most parents are happy to get their child to take a medication once or twice a day. However, some children with ASD and/or ADHD do better with clonidine four times daily than other medications. I have had some success with this medication when other treatments have failed, but due to sedation it is not my first or second choice.

Clonidine has the potential of decreasing your child's blood pressure, but this is rarely significant enough to cause a problem. You should notify your physician if your child complains of being dizzy or having vision problems, or if you suspect low blood pressure for any reason. Vital signs, including blood pressure, should be checked at each visit with your pediatrician or child psychiatrist.

A long-acting formulation of clonidine is available, clonidine ER (Kapvay). This is given only twice a day rather than three or four times a day for regular clonidine. This makes getting your child to take the medication much easier, but it can still be sedating for some children. Children are generally much less likely to be sedated if they are also taking a stimulant at the same time (if the stimulant is appropriate for other reasons as well). This medication must be swallowed whole. If it is chewed, it will not be long-acting anymore and your child will get the whole day's dose at once (2).

Another nonstimulant medication is guanfacine, a sort of "cousin" of clonidine. It is in the same medication class as clonidine but is less likely to cause sedation. It also lasts longer than clonidine and can be given less often (it is generally given two or three times per day). For these reasons, it is much preferred over clonidine in clinical practice. The long-acting form (guanfacine ER [Intuniv]) is a once-daily medication and is generally given in the morning. In my clinical experience, this medication is more convenient and less sedating than clonidine or clonidine ER (Kapvay). It is FDA approved for the treatment of ADHD in children and adults, both used alone and in combination with a stimulant. Studies of guanfacine have shown improvements in hyperactivity, inattention, insomnia, and tics in those with ADHD and ASD. Response rates in these different studies ranged from 24% to 58%, especially for hyperactivity. Studies of guanfacine ER (Intuniv) have also shown improvements in irritability in those with ASD. Possible side effects are irritability, sedation, sleep disturbances, constipation, headache, and bedwetting. This medication has a relatively benign side effect profile. A randomized, double-blind, placebo-controlled trial of guanfacine ER showed effectiveness in controlling

ADHD symptoms in those with ASD, especially patients with hyperactivity (2,5).

One of my preferred combinations for children with ADHD and ASD is long-acting methylphenidate (Concerta) and guanfacine ER (Intuniv). Using Intuniv with another stimulant, besides methylphenidate ER, is also quite effective. This combination treatment for ADHD is increasingly common and seems to work quite well in many children for control of inattention, impulsivity, hyperactivity, and sometimes even anger outbursts. Although not likely, I have had cases in which the addition of Intuniv prevented the need to add risperidone (Risperdal) for tantrums and aggression. Furthermore, since the Intuniv dose lasts for 24 hours, it offers some control of ADHD symptoms when the stimulant has worn off in the afternoon. Without the Intuniv, the child would have no control of ADHD symptoms after midafternoon. Thus, Intuniv can help make family time in the late afternoon and evenings better as the child has some control of ADHD symptoms. However, the important thing to note is that the ADHD symptom control with Intuniv is not as much as with the stimulant. Thus, you should not expect complete control of ADHD symptoms during the late afternoon or evening simply because your child is taking Intuniv. The most common side effect from this medication that I see in clinical practice is midafternoon drowsiness in a minority of children. In very few cases, this is problematic enough that it requires stopping the medication. Intuniv is generally very well tolerated. Do not be surprised or upset if your child's doctor recommends a combination treatment. It is likely to work quite well. But not all children with ADHD and ASD will need this combination.

Atomoxetine (Strattera) is a different type of nonstimulant altogether. It is a selective norepinephrine reuptake inhibitor that is FDA approved for ADHD in children and adults.

It is not a blood pressure medication, as are the previous nonstimulants. Strattera is moderately effective for the treatment of hyperactivity and possibly inattention in those with ASD. One study showed a 60% response rate with improvements in conduct, hyperactivity, learning, and inattention. Another study showed a 75% response rate with additional improvements in irritability, social withdrawal, stereotypy, and repetitive speech. Side effects from atomoxetine are irritability, decreased appetite, mood swings, gastrointestinal symptoms, sleep problems, ear ringing, and sedation. The most common side effects are fatigue, nausea, and decreased appetite (2). This medication is not typically prescribed as the first medication trial by most physicians but probably works quite well in a certain proportion of those with ASD. It has been shown to be especially helpful in patients with anxiety and ADHD symptoms. Generally, the response is not as high as with stimulants, and it takes 2 to 4 weeks to notice significant improvement with this medication. Interestingly, a study evaluating longer-term efficacy found that the medication continued to grow in effectiveness even 6 months after starting the medication. If your child cannot tolerate stimulants, this is a good medication choice. There is also evidence that this medication can decrease anxiety to some degree as well (2,5).

OTHER MEDICATIONS THAT MAY BE USED OFF-LABEL FOR ADHD

Often medications that have been FDA approved for a particular purpose or for a certain age group are still used by physicians to treat other disorders or other age groups. This is called "off-label use." For example, bupropion (Wellbutrin) is FDA approved for the treatment of depression in adults, but it can be used off-label to treat depression in children or to treat another disorder such as ADHD. This can be very appropriate and is still the standard of care.

Bupropion (Wellbutrin) is an antidepressant that has been used off-label to decrease ADHD symptoms, especially in those who are not benefitting enough from or cannot tolerate stimulants or nonstimulants. Its effectiveness is less than that of the stimulants and nonstimulants already discussed.

Although technically not a nonstimulant, at times amantadine is used to treat ADHD and behavioral symptoms. It is an NMDA antagonist and is typically used to treat Parkinsonism and influenza. Although the effect on ASD of this medication is low, it is especially helpful for reducing hyperactivity. It may be considered an option in certain cases but certainly not as a first-line medication. One study showed significant improvements in hyperactivity and inappropriate speech. There have also been studies of this medication being used in combination with an atypical antipsychotic medication (discussed later) to improve tantrums and irritability as well (6).

For completeness, I will mention several other medications that are not typically used solely for ADHD symptoms but that have shown some efficacy in controlling ADHD symptoms. Risperidone (Risperdal) is an atypical antipsychotic that has been shown to be effective in decreasing hyperactivity. In one study, 69% of patients had improvements in hyperactivity. Aripiprazole (Abilify), also an atypical antipsychotic, has shown some mild improvements in hyperactivity as well. However, due the atypical antipsychotics' side-effect profile or potential for producing long-term side effects, they are not likely ever to be used simply to control hyperactivity. The benefits would not likely outweigh the risks for this symptom. Later in this chapter we will discuss this class of medication when we discuss how to control tantrums, irritability, and aggression, as these are FDA approved for this purpose.

Similar to Abilify and Risperdal is haloperidol (Haldol). It is a conventional (first-generation) antipsychotic medication. It also has shown some improvements in reducing hyperactivity, but as it has a higher risk of producing extrapyramidal symptoms (EPS; movement disorders/tics) and long-term side effects, the benefits may not outweigh the risks (1).

Another medication found to produce some improvement in hyperactivity is naltrexone. This medication is used at times to decrease self-injurious behavior such as head-banging or biting. Studies have shown it may help a little with hyperactivity as well. Some studies have also shown that it produces some improvements in executive functioning (judgment). Side effects are sedation, decreased appetite, and vomiting (1).

Whether stimulants or nonstimulants are used, I would strongly recommend that your child's ADHD symptoms and medication effectiveness be monitored regularly by sending forms to teachers so they can gather information. Your physician should give these to you. These forms make your child's ADHD symptoms as objective as possible and allow some way of monitoring for the need to change or adjust medications. How the teachers feel your child is doing is very important because they see your child in what is his or her most difficult and demanding environment. Also, if your child is taking a stimulant medication, the time the medication is taking effect in your child is predominately at school. The teacher would be the best witness as to whether this medication is helpful, and to what degree. Various forms can be used for this purpose, such as Vanderbilt forms or SNAP forms. You can even get SNAP forms online for free. If you do not use specific forms, bring as much written or verbal feedback from teachers as possible to the appointment so that your child's doctor can determine whether or not medication adjustments are needed. Especially bring any discipline notes to the appointments.

In summary, the nonstimulants are generally not as effective as the stimulants in treating your child's ADHD symptoms. However, they can be very helpful when used along with a stimulant (if needed) to maximize treatment of ADHD symptoms or when stimulants cannot be tolerated. They can also be helpful in the treatment of tics. The nonstimulants generally are more helpful in treating hyperactivity and impulsivity than inattention. However, the side effects from nonstimulants are quite different from those of stimulants, making them potentially more tolerable for your child. There are many different medication options to treat your child's ADHD symptoms. Do not give up. Although for most children the first medication works and is a good fit, it may take more than one or even several trials to find the best medication for your child. Be honest about your concerns with your child's doctor, and report any side effects.

ATYPICAL (SECOND-GENERATION) ANTIPSYCHOTIC MEDICATIONS

The only two medications that have so far been approved by the FDA specifically for those with ASD are risperidone (Risperdal) and aripiprazole (Abilify). Risperdal was approved in 2006, Abilify in 2009. Both medications are available in generic forms now. Risperdal is FDA approved starting at age 5 and Abilify at age 6. However, your doctor may treat at earlier ages, depending on severity of symptoms. Your doctor will always weigh the risks and benefits of medications, making sure that the benefits outweigh the risks. This includes the consideration of how young to treat and whether or not prescribing a medication off-label (outside of FDA approval parameters of age and diagnosis) is appropriate. Sometimes it may be reasonable to treat with these medications earlier than their FDA-approved ages. Risperdal and Abilify are specifically approved for the treatment of impairing irritability, aggression, self-injury, and severe tantrums. These medications have also been shown to improve stereotypy (movements such as hand-flapping and other stereotypical behaviors) and hyperactivity. However, due to the possible metabolic side effects (discussed later), you would not want to use these medications simply for hyperactivity or stereotypies, but these could be added benefits if your child already needs these medications for severe irritability (2,4).

These medications have been extensively studied and shown to be very effective in significantly reducing severe irritability, tantrums, self-injury, and aggression. Unfortunately, these medications do not technically improve the "core" symptoms of ASD such as communication and social impairments. Most parents and experienced providers will tell you, however, that they sometimes note some improvements in communication, eye contact, or socialization upon starting an atypical antipsychotic medication. Although the response is not dramatic, it can still be significant to the parent or child. This may be an indirect effect of the child being less irritable and less overwhelmed on the new medication or a direct effect of the medication. However, you should not expect any specific improvements in the "core" symptoms of ASD, and these medications certainly do not "cure" ASD (2).

In 2007, a systematic review and meta-analysis on the use of Risperdal in children with ASD was published. Significant benefits were found for irritability, social withdrawal, and hyperactivity, and modest decreases were found in inappropriate speech and stereotypies. A study in adults with ASD showed a significant reduction in self-injurious behavior. The most common side effects were increased appetite, somnolence, drowsiness, fatigue, nasal congestion, enuresis (urinary incontinence), dry mouth, diarrhea, and constipation. In 2012, the same group published a systematic review and meta-analysis on Abilify and found results similar to those mentioned above for Risperdal (4).

One study that led to the FDA's approval of Risperdal for irritability in children with ASD showed a 69% response rate with a 57% decrease in irritability. Doses in the study ranged from 0.5 to 3.5 mg per day, with an average dose of about 2 mg per day. A study in adults showed improvement in aggression, irritability, anxiety, depression, and repetitive behaviors, with a 57% response rate. The doses in this study ranged from 1 to 10 mg per day. Thus, there is good evidence that risperidone is associated with significant improvements in various symptoms associated with ASD (5).

Short-term studies (8 weeks) and long-term studies (52 weeks) have shown that Abilify can be effective in reducing irritability in those with ASD. Dosages for Abilify in these studies ranged from 2.5 to 15 mg per day (4,7). One study found that it was generally safe and well tolerated even after 1 year, but abnormalities were noted in lipids/cholesterol and blood sugar levels, on average. For example, there was a 5% increase in cholesterol and a 2% increase in blood sugar. About 10% of those in the study discontinued Abilify secondary to side effects of weight gain or aggression. Even after 52 weeks, irritability remained improved, however. Therefore, there is strong evidence that aripiprazole (Abilify) is effective in reducing irritability and tantrums in the long term, although blood sugar and cholesterol levels need to be monitored (4).

Being a parent of a child with ASD, I can certainly attest that the most impairing and disruptive symptom of ASD is often irritability, especially with tantrums, aggression, or self-injury. The quality of life for the child with ASD who has severe irritability can dramatically improve with the use of this class of medications. Some examples of children who could benefit from such a medication are those who have such severe irritability that they cannot participate or learn in class; those who cannot tolerate socialization and are easily overwhelmed by minor changes in routine to the point of tantrums; those who engage in frequent self-injurious behavior; and those who have significant aggression directed toward caregivers and/or peers. With appropriate use of an atypical antipsychotic, your child may be able to participate more fully in class and in therapies. There is no doubt that this has the potential to change the trajectory of your child's life, especially when used at early, crucial stages in a child's life. However, the decision of whether or not to use an atypical antipsychotic should be handled on an individual basis, taking many factors into account. Only you and your doctor can decide whether this medication is right for your child, especially weighing potential long-term risks. But you should not be afraid to use this medication if your doctor decides it is appropriate for your child.

The ability of these medications to decrease irritability and significantly improve functioning can be a sort of "miracle" for your family and child. For example, with this medication, your family life can change from dealing with severe tantrums multiple times per day that last up to 40 minutes to only one or two tantrums per week, lasting 10 minutes at a time. Of course, results vary from child to child. Your child may go from a self-contained classroom to a regular education classroom because of improvements in behavior. Your child is likely to be able to learn now and improve at a more rapid pace since his or her behaviors are under better control. Treatment with these medications can sometimes allow your family to go from being unable to leave the home because of your child's severe tantrums to being able to go to the store, restaurants, or vacations together.

Risperidone's effect on reducing irritability has been shown to be maintained with long-term use. Also, a recent study showed that a combination of parent training and risperidone was more effective than only risperidone. For this reason, you should consider parenting skills training along with this medication. This parent training includes education on ASD and how to better manage your child's difficult behavior. Often this type of training is included in ABA therapy as well (2).

A small study comparing aripiprazole (Abilify) to risperidone (Risperdal) in children with ASD showed that both medications produce comparable improvements in terms of decreasing problem behaviors. The side effects were also similar, including the amount of weight gain. Thus, either one of these medications is a good choice if your doctor recommends it for your child's behavioral symptoms. However, in clinical experience, weight gain seems to be less with aripiprazole (Abilify), while risperidone (Risperdal) seems to work a little better on average than aripiprazole for problem behaviors in those with ASD. I mention this so that you understand that it is common practice to start with risperidone, due to its good effectiveness and cheaper cost, but then change to aripiprazole if risperidone is ineffective or there is too much weight gain from risperidone. Weight gain is quite common, so this is very important. You should not give up on this entire class of medication simply because of weight gain. You should try another medication, such as Abilify or others (2,8).

Olanzapine (Zyprexa) is another atypical antipsychotic found to improve behaviors in those with ASD. However, it is not FDA approved for use in ASD. Also, since it causes even more weight gain than risperidone (on average), it is rarely used. There are generally better choices that are associated with less weight gain (2).

Although there are numerous other atypical antipsychotics, they are not FDA approved for ASD and, more importantly, there are not any "good studies" (randomized, double-blind, placebo-controlled trials) showing their effectiveness in treating ASD- associated behavioral problems. Other atypical antipsychotics are quetiapine (Seroquel), ziprasidone (Geodon), paliperidone (Invega), iloperidone (Fanapt), asenapine (Saphris), cariprazine (Vraylar), and lurasidone (Latuda). They may be used as third-line agents by your provider if your child fails to respond to trials of risperidone and/or aripiprazole. It is not uncommon to use these medications if a child gains too much weight from risperidone or aripiprazole, or if these medications have been ineffective for your child. Also, although it is off-label use, these medications are still in the same class as the FDA-approved medications, and they may be effective for your child. Do not be afraid to follow the directions of your provider, but be informed. Ask why your child's provider is prescribing an off-label medication (2,5).

Because aripiprazole and ziprasidone are generally regarded as the most "weight-neutral" medications in their class of atypical antipsychotics, ziprasidone (Geodon) is often used in practice when a child is gaining too much weight while taking risperidone or even aripiprazole. I have had success in treating children and adults for irritability and tantrums with ziprasidone with less weight gain than with risperidone. But there have not been any large randomized, double-blind, placebo-controlled trials of ziprasidone for ASD. As a result, you should probably not use ziprasidone as a first-line medication because there is less evidence regarding its effectiveness.

One small study showed quetiapine was poorly tolerated and minimally effective in children with ASD. In small studies, paliperidone and ziprasidone appeared promising, but more studies are needed (2,9).

Haloperidol (Haldol) is a first-generation antipsychotic. It improves behavior symptoms in the short term and long term, but with more risk of extrapyramidal symptoms and tardive dyskinesia. These are essentially drug-induced movement disorders. One study showed that by 6 months, 34% of children had developed a dyskinesia (movement disorder). Female gender, length of treatment, and dosage strength increased the risk of the dyskinesias. Sedation was also a side effect. The dosages in these studies ranged from 0.5 to 4 mg per day. Risperdal was shown in one study to work for a broader range of behaviors with less risk of these side effects. Risperdal was superior to Haldol in improving behavioral symptoms, language skills, social relations, and impulsivity (2). Furthermore, one study showed no difference in weight gain between Haldol and Risperdal, meaning there would not even be the benefit of less weight gain when using Haldol to treat irritability in those with ASD. If your physician recommends Haldol in place of risperidone, you should ask a lot of questions. It is less expensive but not as effective, and it likely has more side effects (4–6).

I have learned from numerous cases to never give up and to never quit searching for options for my patients. I have had several patients who did not respond well enough to several medications tried. After responding very poorly to many medications, one patient finally responded very well to the fifth atypical antipsychotic tried. Her life is now far better and she is much more functional, no longer being held back by her severe tantrums and irritability. Thus, as the parent, you should never give up either. This is why I have included seemingly more information than some parents might want to know about medications. You need to know that there are many options. Although your child is likely to respond to the first medication given, you may have to be patient and try numerous medications before finding the right fit. Do not give up if your child fails to respond to trials of risperidone and aripiprazole. Try some of the other atypical antipsychotics. My preferred other atypical antipsychotics are ziprasidone and paliperidone. There have been some promising studies with these medications.

There can be many risks associated with an atypical antipsychotic medication. First, you need to be aware that the weight gain can be quite significant. I see in my practice 0 to 2 lbs of weight gain per month in children, which can certainly add up over time. Rarely, the rate of weight gain can be higher, such as 4 lbs per month, but it typically levels off after time, but sometimes only after many months or years. If the child started off thin or underweight, it could take a while for this to be worrisome. If the child is already overweight, however, this can be a problem quickly. Some studies have shown that those taking an atypical antipsychotic for the first time, younger patients, and those with a higher starting weight were more susceptible to weight gain while taking these medications (2).

We do not yet have a great solution for the problem of weight gain with these medications. If a patient gains too much weight, I may switch from risperidone to aripiprazole or ziprasidone, as these medications are likely to cause less weight gain and may be just as effective. Another option is adding topiramate (Topamax), an antiseizure medication that is commonly used in low doses for migraines or weight loss in adults. This can help decrease appetite and weight. In some cases, topiramate can cause word-finding problems or numbness or tingling in the extremities, so you will want to monitor for these as side effects.

Another option is to see an endocrinologist and have the child placed on metformin, a diabetes medication that is known to help prevent diabetes and lower weight. Although the most obvious option is a very healthy diet and a sound exercise plan to help decrease the weight of those taking an atypical antipsychotic, it is not as easy as one would hope. The atypical antipsychotics do affect metabolism and appetite. Furthermore, children with ASD are often picky eaters secondary to sensory integration problems (food texture aversions) and insistence on sameness (same routine diet). You should get a consultation with a nutritionist, who may be able to offer solutions. Also, try to find ways to increase your child's activity level.

Other than weight gain, there is the risk of increasing cholesterol/lipids and blood sugar levels when taking an atypical antipsychotic. As a result of these risks, your doctor should obtain a sample of your child's blood (fasting) before or soon after starting the medication, again in 3 months, and then every 6 months thereafter to monitor for these side effects. Typically when blood sugar and/or lipid levels do increase, they slowly creep up over time, often over many years. Thus, the real short-term side effect is weight gain. The majority of patients I treat do not have significant increases in blood sugar or cholesterol levels. It appears that this side effect is very individual and unpredictable. For example, there are rare cases of an increase in the blood sugar level within 3 months, while others have no significant changes in blood sugar or cholesterol levels over 10 years. The metabolic side effects or changes in these numbers can be independent of weight gain. Thus, even if your child is not gaining weight, his or her blood sugar or cholesterol levels could still be increasing.

Extrapyramidal symptoms, such as dystonia (muscle cramp) or muscle rigidity or tics, are possible as more immediate side effects. If your child is taking an atypical antipsychotic and gets a sudden, painful muscle cramp, you should use over-the-counter diphenhydramine (Benadryl) to quickly reverse this side effect. These side effects are unusual and reversible but can happen shortly after starting the medication. Do not expect these to happen, but if they do, call your doctor.

Tardive dyskinesia is an extrapyramidal symptom (movement disorder) that presents rarely and after taking this type of medication for many years. The risk of tardive dyskinesia increases with the dose and the length of time taking the medication. The risk is very low with the newer atypical (second-generation) antipsychotics such as Risperdal, Abilify, and others. Tardive dyskinesia was more common when the older (first-generation) antipsychotics were used, such as haloperidol (Haldol). Although tardive dyskinesia is rare, it is worth weighing this risk before starting this type of medication, since it can be irreversible.

Gynecomastia (growing breasts in males) is a potential side effect of any medication in this class, but the risk is greater with risperidone. The risk is still quite low, but if you notice anything abnormal with your child's chest, tell your doctor. Unfortunately, gynecomastia is not uncommon even during normal puberty without an antipsychotic. Gynecomastia can be reversible in some cases, especially if caught early.

Lastly, there is a risk of galactorrhea with the use of antipsychotic medications. This is inappropriate lactation (milk production from the breasts) and is caused by an increase of the hormone prolactin that can occur with the use of some antipsychotics. The risk of galactorrhea is low but depends on which antipsychotic is used and the dosage. Galactorrhea can occur in 20% to 25% of women even if they are not taking an antipsychotic. There are other medications and numerous medical causes as well. This side effect can be quite bothersome or disturbing, but it is reversible upon the discontinuation of the antipsychotic, although it can take weeks or months for it to resolve completely. Your child can also be changed to another antipsychotic medication that is much less likely to cause this.

The above is not an exhaustive list of side effects associated with the use of antipsychotic medications to help with ASD, but it does include the most relevant ones. Discuss any other concerns with your doctor.

Specific monitoring schedules are recommended when using an antipsychotic medication such as Abilify or Risperdal. This may help you feel comfortable in knowing that your doctor is ordering all of the necessary laboratory tests and studies. It is recommended that baseline body-mass index (BMI) measurements be taken initially and at follow-up appointments. Monitoring protocols for metabolic changes vary considerably, but most experts recommend obtaining baseline blood levels of fasting blood sugar, hemoglobin A1c, fasting lipids, liver function tests, prolactin, and thyroid stimulating hormone (TSH). Most physicians will also get a complete metabolic profile, which also gives information regarding kidney function, electrolytes, and so forth. They also typically will get a complete blood count (CBC) to test for anemia and neutropenia (low levels of a particular white blood cell) as well as other problems in the blood. Follow-up testing should especially be done for fasting blood sugar and lipid levels. Most physicians also include hemoglobin A1c in this follow-up blood work, as it is the best predictor of the person's blood sugar levels over the last 3 months. It is generally recommended to get follow-up blood tests after the first 3 months on the medication and then every 6 months. Your child's doctor will likely monitor prolactin levels only if there are physical signs or symptoms of elevation present. Your doctor will know to look for these signs and symptoms. As many children have low vitamin D levels, I also check at least initial vitamin D levels. A low vitamin D level is known to have an effect on mood and behavior, as well as metabolism (7).

SELECTIVE SEROTONIN REUPTAKE INHIBITORS

SSRIs are medications that increase the levels of serotonin in the brain. SSRIs are approved for many purposes in adults but are not specifically approved for adults with ASD. SSRIs are approved for adults who have OCD, generalized anxiety disorder, major depressive disorder, premenstrual dysphoric disorder, social anxiety disorder, panic disorder, and posttraumatic stress disorder. In children, fluoxetine (Prozac) is approved for treating OCD and depression, while fluvoxamine (Luvox) and sertraline (Zoloft) are only approved for treating OCD. Escitalopram (Lexapro) is approved for use in teenagers with depression. Thus, if your child with ASD has any of these comorbidities, one of these SSRIs may be recommended by your doctor. Preferably your physician would use one of the SSRIs that is FDA approved for your child's specific age and disorder, whenever possible.

Although there is not a specific indication or FDA approval for children with ASD, it was assumed (and hoped) that SSRIs would be helpful for the OCD-like symptoms and repetitive behaviors often associated with ASD. Thus, many physicians have used SSRIs to treat repetitive behaviors or mental rigidity in children with ASD. This also includes insistence on sameness, the need for routine, and rituals. Unfortunately, these symptoms are apparently not similar enough to "true" OCD for the SSRIs to work for these behaviors or symptoms in children with ASD. In fact, studies have clearly shown that SSRIs, especially fluoxetine (Prozac) and fluvoxamine (Luvox), are not effective for these symptoms in children, although they have some efficacy in reducing these behaviors in adults. Given this evidence, it is not appropriate to use SSRIs simply for repetitive behaviors or insistence on sameness in children with ASD. They may be helpful in adults with ASD for repetitive behaviors and insistence on sameness. SSRIs may still be appropriate for your child with ASD if there are other comorbidities present, such as severe anxiety, depression, or OCD (2,5,6).

Despite numerous studies indicating that the most common comorbid disorder in children with ASD is anxiety, there are no high-quality studies addressing medication treatment of this specifically in children with ASD (1). However, SSRIs are commonly prescribed in practice for significant anxiety in those with ASD as there are numerous studies validating SSRI use to treat anxiety disorders in children without ASD. A secondary reason to treat anxiety in your child with ASD is that anxiety can increase behavioral problems (7). Thus, it is important that it be recognized and treated for more reasons than the anxiety itself. Anxiety can also lead to more social withdrawal, and this would exacerbate your child's avoidance and preference to be alone. In my experience, it is not uncommon for individuals with ASD, especially those who are higher functioning, to become depressed or have social anxiety disorder. This is likely a result of greater awareness of their differences or more recognition of bullying.

The most likely anxiety disorders in those with ASD are simple phobias, generalized anxiety disorder, separation anxiety disorder, and OCD (1). Anxieties and phobias are found in up to 50% of children with ASD. Some studies indicate that OCD is the second most common comorbid condition with ASD, after ADHD, with more than one third of patients continuing to have obsessions or compulsions that limit their ability to interact socially (10). In practice, however, it is sometimes difficult to sort out circumscribed interests from obsessions. Thus, you may feel that a circumscribed interest is an obsession, but if it is truly not bothersome to your child and is enjoyable, it is a circumscribed interest. A circumscribed interest is unlikely to respond to an SSRI. Obsessions are bothersome and not enjoyable and might respond to an SSRI. Other studies have shown that social anxiety disorder is prevalent as well. This can also be effectively treated with an SSRI.

In adults with ASD, both fluoxetine (Prozac) and fluvoxamine (Luvox) have shown improvements (about 50% response rate) in repetitive behaviors and thoughts, aggression, and other behavioral problems. In one small study of adults with ASD, sertraline (Zoloft) improved self-injurious behavior and aggression in eight of nine subjects. Sertraline has been found to be moderately effective and relatively well tolerated in decreasing repetitive behaviors and aggression in adults with ASD (5).

Other types of antidepressant medications that could be used by your provider include tricyclic antidepressants. However, so far these have been shown to cause too many side effects, and there is insufficient evidence to support their use. Another class is the serotonin and norepinephrine reuptake inhibitors (SNRIs). Although there are no data on the use of SNRIs in those with ASD, they are used to treat depression and multiple types of anxiety in adults. Only duloxetine (Cymbalta) has an FDA approval for use in children at all, and this is for children and adolescents with generalized anxiety disorder. Duloxetine may be an option if your child has chronic worry and generalized anxiety disorder.

ANTIEPILEPTIC (ANTICONVULSANT) DRUGS

There are multiple medications falling into the category of anticonvulsants that are used for seizure disorders and mood and behavioral disorders. The most commonly used medications in this class for psychiatric purposes are oxcarbazepine (Trileptal), carbamazepine (Tegretol), topiramate (Topamax), valproate (Depakote), and lamotrigine (Lamictal). The medications in this class can often be used for multiple problems. One such example is the use of topiramate (Topamax) for seizures, mood stabilization, weight loss, migraine prevention, and so forth. Overall, however, the results from studies using antiepileptic medications for better control of behavior, irritability, and other symptoms associated with ASD have been disappointing. However, for many years some physicians have used this class of medication as they produce fewer side effects than atypical antipsychotics and intuitively should have worked in those children with ASD. Your physician may still recommend this class of medications for the above reasons, but you should know that the evidence does not support their effectiveness. If your child does not respond well to atypical antipsychotics or has too many side effects, then an antiepileptic medication may be worth a trial.

GLUTAMATERGIC AND GAMMA-AMINOBUTYRIC ACIDERGIC AGENTS

Changes in glutamatergic (excitatory) and gamma-aminobutyric acid (inhibitory) neurotransmissions have been implicated in ASD. Many scientists hope that medications that work on these specific chemicals may be the answer to finally improving the actual core symptoms of ASD (2).

A small but good-quality study of N-acetylcysteine (NAC) showed improvements in irritability in children with ASD. However, other NMDA receptor antagonists, such as amantadine, memantine (Namenda), and riluzole, failed to show effectiveness in high-quality studies. More recently, small good-quality trials showed improvements with amantadine, memantine, riluzole, and NAC, each in combination with risperidone. These medications may be significantly effective only if taken along with risperidone. Thus, your physician may use these medications in combination with risperidone to more effectively treat your child's behavioral symptoms (2,4,8).

Memantine (Namenda), an Alzheimer's dementia medication, has shown a 61% response rate in children and adolescents with ASD in one small study (18 subjects). Improvements were noted in social withdrawal and inattention. Another study (151 children and young adults) showed some improvements in language, social behavior, and self-stimulatory stereotypic behaviors. However, all of these studies were not of high enough quality to recommend this medication for regular use. More studies are needed. Your physician may recommend this medication as there is a growing evidence base for its use in ASD, especially for behavioral symptoms and language (2).

CHOLINERGIC AGENTS

Two studies of donepezil (Aricept), used commonly for Alzheimer's patients, showed mixed results. One study indicated improvement in language, while the other did not. The quality of the studies was low, so more studies are needed. I mention this medication because this class of medications is being used more often recently in those with ASD (2,6).

OXYTOCIN

Oxytocin is a natural chemical in the pituitary gland involved in newborn attachment, uterine contractions, and milk letdown. There are multiple studies under way, and it is hoped that oxytocin may improve social behavior and social communication in ASD populations. Studies in adults and adolescents have indicated improvements in eye contact and social learning. Data will be available on this within the next few years. Based on studies so far, it may be that it can be administered before therapy sessions to enhance social learning (2,4).

OTHER AGENTS

Some have postulated that dysfunction in the natural opiate system may cause sensory disturbances and self-injurious behaviors. Possibly, higher levels of circulating natural opiates cause lower pain sensation and corresponding self-injurious behaviors. Naltrexone, an opioid antagonist, is a medication that is sometimes used clinically to decrease these behaviors. Studies indicate possible improvement in hyperactivity and restlessness, but there is no clear evidence of a decrease in the core symptoms of ASD. This medication may be prescribed by your physician if your child has self-injurious behavior. It is generally well tolerated but can cause nausea (2,6).

Omega-3 fatty acids (fish oil) have been studied to see if there were improvements in ASD or ADHD symptoms, but the only symptom reduction occurred in hyperactivity, and only to a mild degree. However, given that this is an over-the-counter product and is thought to be important for overall physical health anyway, it is worth a trial (2).

The most studied agent in ASD is secretin. In 16 high-quality studies, it was not found to be effective in treating the core symptoms of ASD and should not be used.

SLEEP

Sleep disturbances are quite common in children with ASD. They may occur in up to 75% to 80% of children with neurodevelopmental disorders. Impaired sleep may cause physical problems but also predisposes children to mood, behavioral, and cognitive impairments. There is clear evidence that poor sleep adversely affects memory, learning, cognitive flexibility, attention, verbal creativity, abstract reasoning, and other executive functions. Poor sleep is also known to result in increased irritability, poor affect modulation, depression, impulsivity, hyperactivity, and aggressiveness. Other health outcomes of inadequate sleep in children include potential negative effects on cardiovascular, immune, and various metabolic systems. This includes problems with glucose metabolism and endocrine functions. There is also an increase in impaired coordination and in accidental injuries (11).

Sleep hygiene is very important. If your child is having difficulty sleeping, you should first make sure you and your child are practicing good sleep hygiene. Pay attention to environmental characteristics such as temperature, noise level, amount of light, incentives to staying up (such as electronics in the room [TV, tablet, videogames, etc.]), and other features that might make it difficult for your child to sleep. Having "screen time" before bed also appears to disrupt sleep patterns. It is best to have your child read or be read to before bed, but you should not do the reading in bed. Your child should use his or her bed only for sleep. Sleep scheduling is also very important. Your child should go to sleep and wake up at the same time each day. This promotes establishment of a regular sleep cycle/pattern. Establishment of a clear bedtime routine helps to cue your child's mind for sleep. This is probably more important for children with ASD, as they need more routine. Thus, having a clear and consistent evening routine is important. This may include taking a bath/shower, brushing teeth, and reading before bed. You should also try to make sure your child gets regular exercise and does not eat too late. Avoid any caffeine in the afternoon and evening, including chocolate. Exercise during the day is also important to decrease hyperactivity before bed (11).

Improving sleep hygiene practices should always be tried first, but if your child's sleep fails to improve with these changes, you doctor may consider medication. The evidence base supports the use of melatonin. Melatonin is the only compound that has been subjected to a controlled study to determine its effectiveness in treating insomnia in those with ASD. One study showed that the children fell asleep on average 51 minutes sooner and slept about 1 hour longer after taking melatonin. Other agents that may be used in clinical practice to help with your child's sleep are trazodone, mirtazapine, clonazepam, diphenhydramine (Benadryl), and clonidine (1). I avoid the use of potentially addictive substances such as clonazepam (a benzodiazepine). Typically, after sleep hygiene changes have failed, I will start with melatonin at a dose of 1 to 6 mg, although some studies have gone up to 10 mg. If this is not effective, I may use clonidine or trazodone. Clonidine is a blood pressure medication that usually has little significant effect on blood pressure at low doses, but it helps decrease ADHD symptoms, especially hyperactivity, while causing drowsiness to help your child sleep. Trazodone is an antidepressant, but used in low doses it mainly works to cause drowsiness. Sometimes this is the best medication to use in a child who has trouble both falling asleep and staying asleep. Mirtazapine is also an antidepressant, but I avoid it because it causes weight gain—unless this effect is desired, such as when the child is losing weight while taking a stimulant or for other reasons.

PHARMACOGENETIC TESTING

Pharmacogenetic testing is now available by multiple companies. Your doctor may or may not participate in this, but these tests are being increasingly used to find the best possible medication for your child. Typically, your doctor will take a swab of the inside of your child's cheek and then send it off to a company for testing. Certain markers are then identified from your child's DNA to identify which medications your child is most likely to respond well to and which medications may need a lower or higher dose. Although this sounds amazing (and it can be), it is not a perfect science yet. I have not been as impressed as I had hoped. For example, the test may show that your child will do well with all of the available stimulants, but then when a stimulant medication is tried, he or she may become too irritable while taking it. I think that this test can be a valuable tool, and I would definitely use it if your insurance covers it well (you do not have to pay much for it) or if you have had trouble finding the right medication for your child. In some cases, it can take a while to find the right medication without this test, and this test might reduce some of the trial-and-error that can be involved. I am sure that subsequent pharmacogenetics tests will continue to improve as our knowledge of genetics advances.

CONCLUSION

Although not all children with ASD need to take a medication, many could likely benefit from one. It is up to you and your doctor to decide what is best for your child. I would encourage you to at least have an initial evaluation with a provider such as a child and adolescent psychiatrist or developmental pediatrician to determine what symptoms could be improved with medications. Remember, you do not have to use a medication if you are not comfortable with it. If you try a medication for your child and you do not like it, you can discuss stopping it with your physician. It does not hurt to investigate your child's options. Ask other parents or providers in the autism community whom they would recommend for medication management.

REFERENCES

1. Siegel M. Psychopharmacology of autism spectrum disorder: evidence and practice. *Child Adolesc Psychiatric Clin North Am.* 2012;21:957–973.
2. Ji N, Findling RL. An update on pharmacotherapy for autism spectrum disorder in children and adolescents. *Curr Opin Psychiatry.* 2015;28:91–101.
3. Spencer D, Marshall J, Post B, et al. Psychotropic medication use and polypharmacy in children with autism spectrum disorders. *Pediatrics.* 2013;132(5):833–840.
4. Baribeau DA, Anagnostou E. An update on medication management of behavioral disorders in autism. *Curr Psychiatry Rep.* 2014;16:43.
5. Doyle CA,. McDougle CJ. Pharmacologic treatments for the behavioral symptoms associated with autism spectrum disorders across the lifespan. *Dialogues Clin Neurosci.* 2012;14:263–279.
6. Siegel M, Beaulieu AA. Psychotropic medications in children with autism spectrum disorders: a systematic review and synthesis for evidence-based practice. *J Autism Dev Disord.* 2012;42:1592–1605.
7. Stigler KA. Psychopharmacologic management of serious behavioral disturbance in ASD. *Child Adolesc Psychiatric Clin North Am.* 2014;23:73–82.

8. Tchaconas A, Adesman A. Autism spectrum disorders: a pediatric overview and update. *Curr Opin Pediatr.* 2013;25:130–143.
9. McQuire C, Hassiotis A, Harrison B, Pilling S. Pharmacological interventions for challenging behavior in children with intellectual disabilities: a systematic review and meta-analysis. *BMC Psychiatry.* 2015;15:303.
10. Harrington JW, Allen K. The clinician's guide to autism. *Pediatr Rev.* 2014;35(2):62–113.
11. Jan JE, Owens JA, Weiss MD, Johnson KP, Wasdell MB, Freeman RD, Ipsiroglu OS. Sleep hygiene for children with neurodevelopmental disabilities. *Pediatrics.* 2008;122:1343–1350.
12. Hirota T, Veenstra-VanderWeele J, Hollander E, Kishi T. Antiepileptic medications in autism spectrum disorder: a systematic review and meta-analysis. *J Autism Dev Disord.* 2014;44:948–957.

COMPLEMENTARY AND ALTERNATIVE MEDICINE THERAPIES

Complementary and alternative medicine (CAM) is the collective term used for treatments or therapies that have not typically been part of Western medicine. The "complementary" part of this term means that the treatment may be used along with more conventional medicine, while the "alternative" component of the term implies that it may be used in place of traditional medicine. Most people in the United States choose not to forgo Western medicine and instead combine CAM and conventional medicine, preferring the term "integrative medicine" over "complementary and alternative medicine."

CAM purports to focus on the whole person, including the physical, mental, emotional, and spiritual components of health. A wide variety of treatments can fit under the umbrella of CAM treatments for autism spectrum disorder (ASD). In this chapter, we will discuss many of these treatments and the evidence base for them.

According to studies, 50% to 75% of children with ASD are treated with CAM therapies. Even higher percentages of children with more severe ASD or intellectual disability are treated with CAM. Parents are also more likely to use CAM treatments if the child has seizures, gastrointestinal symptoms, or a behavioral disorder. Parents believe that these therapies are more accessible and less invasive. Most parents are more comfortable when they hear that a treatment falls under the CAM category because they believe it is more "natural" or safer (1,2).

CAM therapies have varying degrees of efficacy and safety data. These different CAM therapies fall under the larger categories of nutrition/dietary interventions, immunomodulation, biochemical and metabolic therapies, detoxification, manipulative and body-based practices, music therapy, sensory integration therapy, hippotherapy (horseback riding), dolphin swim therapy, hyperbaric oxygen therapy, and so forth. It is beyond the scope of this book to discuss each therapy in extensive detail, but I will give an introduction to each type of CAM treatment and then discuss the more important and controversial treatments (2).

1. **Nutrition/dietary interventions** include the gluten-free/ casein-free diet, vitamin C, vitamin B6 and magnesium, carnosine, omega-3 fatty acids, and combined vitamin therapies.

2. **Immunomodulation** includes antibiotic treatments and/or antifungal treatments and the use of probiotics or prebiotics. These are based on the theory that ASD is caused by or exacerbated by problems with the child's immune system or fungal overgrowths. There is no evidence for the use of antifungals for ASD in the literature, and it is likely that long-term antifungal use has many side effects. Some of the known possible side effects from the short-term use of antifungals are nausea, diarrhea, rashes, hair loss, etc. More rarely, lowered immune

system function (low white blood cells), seizures, and liver failure could occur.

3. **Biochemical and metabolic therapies** include precursors and coenzyme factor treatments. These treatments were started secondary to the belief that dysfunctions in several metabolic pathways are involved in ASD. Some chemicals thought to help decrease such abnormalities in metabolism are trimethyl glycine, dimethyl glycine, and vitamin B12 injections.

4. **Detoxification** is based on the belief that ASD is due to heavy metal poisoning. Typically, your child's hair or blood is tested. Unfortunately, these tests are unregulated, and often the person running the test advises chelation therapy to remove the heavy metals. Deaths have occurred from improper chelation protocols. Chelation therapy will be discussed in further detail later in this chapter.

5. **Manipulative and body-based practices** include craniosacral massage, chiropractic manipulation, massage therapy, and therapeutic touch.

6. **Sensory integration therapy** includes some techniques used in occupational therapy but mostly includes the use of auditory integrative therapy to retrain your child's auditory reflexes.

7. **Music and other expressive therapies** use music and art, drama, and other activities to improve a variety of skills.

There are numerous CAM treatments available for ASD, but there is little evidence for most of them. Some of these are likely harmless and potentially helpful, while others could be dangerous. The following sections of this chapter will discuss in greater detail some of the more important and/or controversial CAM treatments. You will undoubtedly come across these CAM treatments and have to make a decision as to whether or not you will use them. This chapter's purpose is to arm you with the proper information you need to make the best, well-informed decision for you and your child.

GLUTEN-FREE/CASEIN-FREE DIET

Arguably, the most commonly discussed CAM treatments are dietary interventions. Data suggest that 15% to 38% of children with ASD use dietary interventions (3). The gluten-free/casein-free (GFCF) diet is the most popular. Gluten is a protein found in wheat, barley, and rye, while casein is a protein found in milk and dairy products. It has been proposed that children with ASD have a "leaky gut" and that they poorly digest casein and gluten. As a result, these proteins (or derivatives of them) allegedly pass into the bloodstream and to the brain, attaching to opioid receptors and thereby causing behavioral, attentional, and physical symptoms. It is thought that the GFCF diet can improve the ASD symptoms and gastrointestinal symptoms (constipation, diarrhea, etc.).

There has been some anecdotal evidence of improvements in children who follow this diet. However, larger double-blind studies have not shown any improvements in attention, sleep, activity, or bowel habits. Only the more poorly designed studies have showed any improvements.

A recent well-designed study evaluated the safety and effectiveness of the GFCF diet. Fourteen children with ASD between the ages of 3 and 5 years were studied for 4 to 6 weeks while on the GFCF diet and then were given challenges with gluten and/or casein snacks. There were no changes or effects on physical symptoms, behavior, or ASD symptoms with the diet or with the gluten and casein snack challenges. However, the GFCF diet was found to be safe and well tolerated with nutritional counseling. Unfortunately, it is doubtful that most children on a GFCF diet also receive nutritional counseling (3).

A large concern regarding the GFCF is that most children on the autism spectrum are already very selective or picky eaters. Some children may eat only four or five different foods, usually with gluten or casein in them. Reducing what the child may eat even more by following such a diet could endanger the child's health. For example, removing gluten could reduce the child's intake of fortified grain products, fiber, and B vitamins, while removing dairy further decreases the child's consumption of vitamin D and calcium. Even children without ASD rarely get enough calcium and vitamin D. Thus, this could be quite a problem. Furthermore, the GFCF diet is more expensive, time-consuming, and likely bothersome to the whole family.

If you decide to try this diet, do not stay on it unnecessarily. If there is no improvement, then stop the diet. Also, please follow up with a nutritionist to make sure it is done in a healthy way. Depriving your child, and his or her brain, of important vitamins and nutrients could do more harm than good. Many parents of children whom I treat feel that they have to "at least try the diet." They do not want to regret not doing it and do not want to leave any stone unturned. In general, even if ineffective, a trial is likely harmless, especially with nutritional guidance. But there is actually good evidence that the diet is not helpful or effective. Even healthcare professionals who believe the diet might be helpful will tell you that it is likely beneficial only in a small subset of children.

OMEGA-3 FATTY ACIDS

It is also common for parents to try omega-3 fatty acids found in fish oil and other products on the market to decrease ASD symptoms. In a randomized, double-blind, placebo-controlled study, a 6-week trial of 1.5 g per day (0.84 g of eicosapentaenoic acid [EPA] and 0.7 g docosahexaenoic acid [DHA]) in 13 children with ASD showed a significant decrease in hyperactivity and stereotypy with no adverse effects. A replication of this study is needed, but certainly as harmless as this supplement should be, it is worth a try. Other studies have shown similar improvements in reducing hyperactivity in those with ADHD without ASD. Some foods with omega-3 fatty acids are mackerel, salmon, cod liver oil, sardines, anchovies, flaxseed, walnuts, chia seeds, and soybeans. Omega-3 comes in multiple forms such as pills, liquids, and gummies, but not all forms have equal amounts of omega-3 or the same ratio of EPA and DHA (some experts believe this ratio is important). I would recommend a trial of this, but discuss it with your child's doctor (1,4,5).

VITAMIN B6

There have been longstanding claims by some that vitamin B6 and magnesium supplementation is helpful. This started in the 1960s when claims were first made that vitamin B6 improved speech and language. The theory underlying potential improvements in those with ASD who took vitamin B6 and magnesium stemmed from the fact that these nutrients are important in the formation of multiple neurotransmitters such as serotonin, dopamine, and norepinephrine. However, a recent review found that there were few studies evaluating the effectiveness of vitamin B6 and magnesium, and of these studies, the sample sizes were small and results were inconclusive. The conclusion of the most recent review was a recommendation against the use of vitamin B6 and magnesium. Furthermore, the long-term use of vitamin B6 has been implicated in sensory peripheral neuropathy (damage to the small nerves in hands and feet), which causes abnormal sensations (1,4).

ARTIFICIAL FOOD COLORS

Artificial food colors (AFCs) are widely used to color beverages and foods. The amount of AFCs that the U.S. Food and Drug Administration has certified has increased more than five-fold, from 12 mg per day per person in 1950 to 68 mg per day per person in 2012. Over the last 40 years, there have been double-blind studies showing adverse behavioral reactions such as hyperactivity in children exposed to AFCs. Studies that used 50 mg or more showed greater behavioral problems in children than studies that used lesser amounts. Although food dyes may increase behavioral problems, there is no evidence that AFCs actually cause ADHD or ASD. As a parent, you should try to at least limit the exposure to food dyes (6).

HYPERBARIC OXYGEN THERAPY

Hyperbaric oxygen therapy (HBOT) uses pressurized oxygen to increase blood flow and oxygen to the brain. This involves inhaling oxygen while sitting in a pressurized chamber (between 1 and 2 atmospheres) for 60 minutes per session. It is thought that this treatment would increase blood flow to the brain, reduce cerebral oxidative stress, and decrease inflammation in the brain. Unfortunately, there are few well-controlled studies regarding this, and HBOT is expensive. The results of the studies that have been done are mixed. The study that showed improvements in behavior, socialization, and language was later found to be quite flawed, and another study that later tried to replicate the findings found no improvements. HBOT is not recommended at this time even by the Undersea and Hyperbaric Medical Society (1,4).

CHEMICAL CHELATION

Chemical chelation has perhaps been the most controversial treatment. It is used especially by those who believe that their child has ASD because of poisoning with heavy metals, such as mercury (see the section on heavy metals in Chapter 4). In two studies, 7% to 8% of parents stated that they had used chelation therapy in their child. There are no well-controlled studies examining the safety or efficacy of chelation, and it has been linked to deaths. A review in 2013 concluded that research does not support the use of chelation for the treatment of ASD. I would advise against this treatment, but if you are contemplating a trial, please discuss with your child's physician (1).

SECRETIN

Secretin, which is often thought of as a CAM treatment, is a natural chemical secreted in the first part of the small intestines that stimulates the release of enzymes from the pancreas and bile from the liver. This would then essentially aid further in digestion. Just as in the case of the GFCF diet, the idea of using secretin as a medicine came from the unproven hypothesis that poor digestion may cause opioid-like peptides to travel to the brain, causing dysfunction. A review of 16 randomized, double-blind, placebo-controlled trials has clearly shown that there is no evidence that secretin is effective in treating the core symptoms of ASD. It is definitely ineffective, and it is expensive (4,5,7).

MELATONIN

Melatonin, which is also technically a CAM treatment, is a hormone produced in the brain by the pineal gland that regulates our circadian rhythms. It has been estimated that about 80% of children with ASD have difficulty with sleep. This includes taking longer to fall asleep, having more nighttime awakenings, and having a decrease in total sleep duration. Melatonin is often given even to typically developing children because it is considered "natural," as well as being inexpensive and available over the counter and having a low side-effect profile. Studies done specifically in children with ASD have found few to no side effects, even with doses of up to 10 mg per night. In one study, 3 of 107 subjects experienced adverse events of bedwetting or feeling groggy in the morning. A large study found that melatonin decreased the time it took for children with ASD to fall asleep and increased the total sleep time by 44 minutes. For most physicians, melatonin is the first medication recommended for children who have significant difficulty with sleep (4).

CANNABIS

Although I would not typically include cannabis even in the CAM category, cannabis is a highly charged political topic that has gained considerable traction in the autism community. For this reason, a thoughtful and evidence-based discussion is warranted. In one study, long-term cannabis use in adolescents (without autism) was associated with a decline in IQ by 5 to 6 points by age 38. Stopping cannabis did not change this decrease in IQ.

The known negative effects of cannabis are as follows:

1. Persistent and nonreversible neurocognitive changes
2. Depression
3. Double the risk of psychosis
4. Impaired brain connections
5. Decreased volumes of brain structures involved in memory, motivation, emotions, and the ability to process emotions

There is no good evidence for cannabis in treating ASD, attention-deficit/hyperactivity disorder (ADHD), and other developmental disabilities. Unfortunately, the use of cannabis for ASD has gained much attention from the traditional media and social media despite the lack of evidence. There has only been a case report of a 6-year-old with ASD who had improvements in hyperactivity, irritability, lethargy, speech impairments, and stereotyped movements. A case report is the lowest form of evidence.

At this point, there is no good evidence that cannabis is helpful and much evidence to support its dangers. Until further research is done, no provider or parent should recommend or use cannabis for autism. If, however, you feel that cannabis may be helpful for autism, support research for it, but definitely do not use it in your child or recommend it to a friend (8).

TIPS ON THE USE OF CAM

As a parent of a child with ASD, you should be wary of any new ASD treatments or fads. There are many people making amazing promises, but they simply want your money. They prey upon us because we are so vulnerable and will do "anything" to help our children. I am not telling you to avoid all new potential treatments, as there may be one that has little research as of yet that might one day work. However, you should not involve your child in a treatment that promises "too much" and is very expensive. You should not give a trial of something that presents a significant health risk with little to no evidence to back up the claim of efficacy. Also, your family resources (especially financial) are precious. Do not spend money you do not have on an empty promise. Discuss any alternative treatment with your doctor first. Your child and your family will need this money in the future. Do not waste money on uncertain treatments when some known evidence-based treatments exist now, such as medications (when appropriate) and Applied Behavior Analysis (ABA) therapy.

Furthermore, it has always struck me as odd that some parents avoid medications or conventional treatments that have clear evidence of safety and efficacy, but they instead prefer CAM treatments that have no established effectiveness and no evidence of safety. Erroneously, parents assume that CAM treatments are safer and more effective even though there is little to no evidence to support this. Some CAM treatments are indeed harmless and slightly effective, such as omega-3 fatty acids or melatonin, while others could be harmful or even deadly. I do not feel that all CAM treatments deserve the "all-natural" and "safe" connotation that they have.

The following guidelines may be helpful when considering CAM treatments for your child:

1. Identify the proposed treatment or therapy.
2. Research the treatment on your own and discuss it with your doctor, being completely honest. Do not hold back out of fear your child's doctor will not agree or will be offended.
3. Learn about the effectiveness and safety of the treatment.
4. Understand exactly what the treatment should improve, such as language, socialization, aggression, behavioral problems, and so forth.
5. Start only one new treatment at a time. If you start more than one, it will be difficult to know to which treatment you should attribute improvements, worsening of problems, or side effects.
6. Understand that your child with ASD will typically have good days and bad days or even good weeks and bad weeks. Thus, do not rapidly attribute a change in behavior to a treatment change. It could be your child's natural variation of his or her behavior/symptoms. If you do this, you may change treatments several times per month without giving anything a fair chance.

7. Be aware of changes in your child's environment that may trigger behavioral problems or regressions.
8. Make sure your child is getting enough sleep. Poor sleep will exacerbate behavioral problems and inattention.
9. If your child suddenly worsens without obvious environmental triggers, make sure he or she is not sick or in pain. Remember that even verbal children with ASD often will not tell you they are in pain or ill. Pain and illness are frequently found to increase aggression, tantrums, or behavioral problems. A frequent cause of behavioral worsening is constipation.
10. Get information about any CAM treatment from multiple sources, including your healthcare professional and even other parents of children with ASD.
11. Understand that even without any treatment, your child is likely to at least slowly improve or move forward developmentally.

It has been recommended that providers consider CAM treatments as follows:

1. If a CAM treatment is safe and effective, then recommend it.
2. If a CAM treatment is safe but the effectiveness is unknown, then tolerate it.
3. If a CAM treatment has a concern for safety but is effective, then monitor closely.
4. If a CAM treatment is unsafe and not effective, then advise against it.

For example, melatonin is considered safe and effective, and thus it would be recommended for a child with insomnia. In contrast, chelation therapy is both unsafe and ineffective, so you should advise against it. Therapies such as massage therapy and dietary supplements are likely safe but should be "tolerated" due to limited information on their effectiveness (2).

These recommendations make sense for parents as well. These recommendations could be roughly translated to parents as follows:

1. If a CAM treatment is safe and effective, then try it.
2. If a CAM treatment is safe but the effectiveness is unknown, then consider it.
3. If a CAM treatment has a concern for safety but is effective, then proceed cautiously with monitoring by a physician.
4. If a CAM treatment is unsafe and not effective, then do not try it.

Ask yourself these questions when deciding on each potential CAM treatment, but always proceed with CAM treatments under a physician's care.

REFERENCES

1. Tchaconas A, Adesman A. Autism spectrum disorders: a pediatric overview and update. *Curr Opin Pediatr.* 2013;25:130–143.
2. Harrington JW, Allen K. The clinician's guide to autism. *Pediatr Rev.* 2014;35(2):62–77.
3. Hyman SL, Stewart PA, Foley J, et al. The gluten-free/casein-free diet: a double-blind challenge trial in children with autism. *J Autism Dev Disord.* 2016;46(1):205–220.
4. Whitehouse AJ. Complementary and alternative medicine for autism spectrum disorders: rationale, safety and efficacy. *J Paediatr Child Health.* 2013;49:E438–442.
5. Ji N, Findling RL. An update on pharmacotherapy for autism spectrum disorder in children and adolescents. *Curr Opin Psychiatry.* 2015;28:91–101.

6. Stevens LJ, Burgess JR, Stochelski MA, Kuczek T. Amounts of artificial food colors in commonly consumed beverages and potential behavioral implications for consumption in children. *Clin Pediatr.* 2014;53(2):133–140.

7. Anagnostou E, Zwaigenbaum L, Szatmari P, et al. Autism spectrum disorder: advances in evidence-based practice. *Can Med Assoc J.* 2014;186(7):509–519.

8. Hadland SE, Knight JR, Harris SK. Medical marijuana: review of the science and implications for developmental-behavioral pediatric practice. *J Dev Behav Pediatr.* 2015;36(2):115–123.

NON-MEDICATION THERAPIES
FOR ASD

There are a multitude of nonpharmacological (non-medication) therapies for autism spectrum disorder (ASD). These therapies generally have mainstream acceptance, especially compared with the complementary and alternative medicine (CAM) treatments mentioned in Chapter 7. Unfortunately, some of these non-medication therapies have little scientific evidence to support their effectiveness. Even those therapies that have some proven efficacy, and likely do work, are based on low-quality studies. Much more research is needed to prove that these therapies improve the symptoms of ASD and associated symptoms, and further studies are needed to differentiate in which children these therapies work best, the necessary treatment frequency and duration, and how young to begin these therapies.

It is paramount that you be vigilant in researching and choosing the best therapy for your child. Many people are more than happy to take your money, and they know that you are vulnerable.

Although many of these non-medication therapies are far from dangerous, wasting your time and money on the wrong therapy is harmful to your child and your family. The younger your child starts therapy or interventions, the greater the improvement is likely to be and the larger the impact on your child's future. Thus, if you waste this window of opportunity on the wrong treatment, you will harm your child's future.

Luckily, there is sound evidence to support some of the therapies we will discuss. Applied Behavioral Analysis (ABA), as well as the behavioral interventions in general, has the best evidence to support its use in improving ASD symptoms in your child.

APPLIED BEHAVIOR ANALYSIS

Behavioral interventions for ASD are the most available and utilized category of nonpharmacological therapies as they are based on learning principles that are quite logical and evidence-based. One of the most widely recognized behavioral interventions/ therapies is ABA, a type of therapy that uses learning and behavior techniques and principles to bring about positive changes in behavior. ABA is effective when applied to academics, adaptive skills, social skills, vocational skills, and communication. The goal of ABA therapy is to increase new skills and decrease problem behaviors. ABA therapy is involved in making behavioral modifications through changes in environmental antecedents (what happened before the behavior) and consequences. Most often, positive reinforcement is used. In the average community, when parents mention behavioral therapy for their child with autism, they are speaking of ABA.

The ABA therapist will perform an initial evaluation and determine in which areas of development your child is behind. The therapist will then develop a plan to reduce interfering behavior (tantrums, aggression, self-injurious behavior, etc.); teach new skills; increase positive behavior; improve social functioning, academics, and self-help skills; increase compliance with tasks; and improve cognitive skills. If your child has difficulty communicating, acquiring new skills, or learning, or is having significant problem behaviors, then ABA is right for your child. ABA therapy is the most evidence-based and most proven therapy for ASD. You should highly consider it for your child.

The ABA therapists often come to your home and will teach you some of these specific skills so that you can better manage problem behaviors and in order to increase the effectiveness of the therapy. The therapist may discuss your child's case with your child's teacher or even go to your child's school to support the teacher and your child through problem behaviors. The therapist will identify triggers in the classroom that the teacher may not notice and develop a plan to improve the child's learning and behaviors in the classroom. Some ABA therapists work in an office setting. In this case, the therapy may be done one on one but not in the home. This may have the benefit of allowing some social interaction with other children undergoing therapy at this office, alternating with one-on-one therapy. The best treatment would likely be a combination of having this therapy at home, at school, and at an office with some social skills training with other peers.

The most evidence-based and well-validated interventions based on ABA principles are Discrete Trials and Pivotal Response Training (PRT). Discrete Trial techniques are regularly included in ABA therapy. PRT also uses some of the same principles of ABA but is less structured than typical ABA therapy.

Discrete Trial Training (DTT) is a way of breaking down learning into smaller parts. It incorporates ABA principles to improve learning and skills development. The steps are as follows: (a) the therapist gains the child's attention, (b) the therapist presents the antecedent intended to elicit the target behavior, (c) the child responds to the stimulus (antecedent) with a particular behavior, (d) the therapist provides a consequence for the behavior, and (e) there is a brief pause before the next trial. The consequence is usually a reinforcement such as giving the child praise, a sticker, or candy for a correct or appropriate behavior. A simple example of DTT is the therapist sitting one on one with a child at a table and trying to teach the child his or her colors:

1. The therapist places one green and one red card on the table in front of John.
2. The therapist states, "Point to the green card."
3. John points to the green card.
4. The therapist states, "Great job!" in an animated voice.
5. There is a pause before the next Discrete Trial begins.

It is important that you understand the basics of DTT because it will be a significant part of your child's ABA therapy and possibly his or her teaching at school. You may even be taught to use DTT with your child at home.

PRT uses similar principles and techniques as ABA but is less structured and more naturalistic. It focuses on specific target skills as well but also core pivotal areas (motivations), which result in gains of joint attention and affect and a decrease in disruptive behavior. PRT seeks to improve responsiveness to treatment, the rate of responding, and affect by allowing child choice and task variation and using direct natural consequences. In other words, the child directs aspects of the therapy based upon his or her interests rather than what the therapist chooses to work on or how the therapist chooses to go about improving a skill. This increases the child's motivation and excitement. A 2014 study that compared a structured ABA approach to PRT found that PRT was more effective at improving social communication skills than the structured ABA. There were greater gains in both the targeted areas and pragmatic skills, stereotyped language, coherence, inappropriate initiation, use of context, and rapport. Thus, the motivational components in PRT proved to be more effective (1). Due to difficulty in studying this therapy directly, researchers have only been able to conclude that it is a "probably efficacious" intervention that cannot be characterized as a "well-established" treatment for ASD (2).

There is evidence that parents who are taught these behavioral principles can apply some of these techniques directly and appropriately without the therapist. Evidence shows that children in parent-directed behavioral programs do make progress, but more progress is made overall when the therapist is directly involved in a regular treatment program. Parents report being more "involved and satisfied" with ABA compared with other therapies or interventions. Parental involvement helps optimize the ABA therapy by having the parent help the therapist to focus on certain problem areas. This involvement also allows the therapist to show the parent more effective and appropriate parenting strategies, individualized to the child. The therapist also serves as an objective party who can identify the child's strengths and weaknesses and formulate a treatment plan (2).

EARLY INTENSIVE BEHAVIORAL INTERVENTION

Early intensive behavioral intervention (EIBI) is a comprehensive therapy based on ABA, or learning theory, principles that seeks to improve expressive and receptive language, imitation, play, joint attention, gross and fine motor skills, and so forth. EIBI also works on decreasing aggression, tantrums, self-injurious behaviors, and vocal or motor stereotypic behavior.

The core features of EIBI are DTT, a 1:1 ratio of adult to child in the early stages of the therapy, and treatment at 20 to 40 hours per week for 1 to 4 years in the school or home setting.

The recommended guidelines are for any therapy for ASD to include the following components: addressing the core symptoms of ASD, a low student–teacher ratio, promotion of family involvement, delivery of therapy in a structured and predictable environment, implementing a functional approach for difficult behaviors, encouraging generalization of what has been learned to the outside world, and monitoring progress over time. All of these characteristics are part of EIBI as well. These guidelines are what you should use when considering a potential program for your child. You should especially make sure the therapist shows you data of your child's behavior and monitors your child's progress over time (3).

This therapy is generally provided for several years at a high intensity and is generally most effective when the child is younger, such as less than 6 years old. A 2012 study found significant improvements in adaptive behavior, receptive language, expressive language, daily communication skills, socialization, and daily living skills. The change in IQ score with the EIBI therapy was about 11 points (3).

One study examined children with ASD upon entry into EIBI therapy and again after 1 year of treatment. They noted that although children older than 2 benefitted from the therapy, those who entered prior to their second birthday did best. Improvements were noted in joint attention, language, imitation, and play. Decreases in stereotypy were also seen. We have known for many years that the earlier the therapy starts, the better the gains on average. Again, this supports early intervention (4).

EIBI is always supervised by a professional trained in ABA procedures and following a treatment manual. Although there is generally improvement in most children with this treatment, it is not clear why some do much better than others. Some characteristics of therapy that may affect treatment outcomes are the treatment/therapy frequency and duration, who provides the treatment, and the intervention setting. The number of months or years that the therapy is used and the number of hours per week probably makes a substantial difference as well. The person providing the service makes a difference, too. It is likely most important that the therapist has a higher level of training and experience, and that the therapist is a clinician rather than a parent or teacher. Also, the goodness of the fit between the therapist and the child intuitively is an important variable. Some of these characteristics of the therapy might even be different depending on the child, or they may affect the child to differing amounts (3). Specifically, studies have shown the most important characteristics of the therapy to be the intensity of the intervention (number of hours per week), the comprehensiveness of the therapy, and the degree of parent involvement (5).

One study of early EIBI found that 86% of mothers and 67% of fathers endorsed practical benefits from the program. These included more support in the home and increased amounts of free time. All parents felt that the parent–child relationship improved, while over half of the parents reported better sibling relationships. Stress levels decreased for 30% of parents (2).

Very little research has been done to evaluate the effectiveness of school-based ABA interventions (ABA therapy delivered only at school). One small study of 11 children (ages 3–7) examined the effectiveness of an "Applied Behavior Analysis (ABA) classroom" educational intervention in a mainstream school setting. The children did quite well with this intervention, learning new skills by the end of 1 year and additional skills by the end of the second year. There were improvements in IQ and adaptive behavior with moderate to large effect sizes. The authors concluded that a comprehensive behavior intervention model could be successfully implemented in a mainstream school setting (6).

It is my belief that without a doubt ABA therapists should be utilized regularly in the classroom. Unfortunately, this is rarely the case despite the fact that there is evidence supporting this, not to mention common sense. Often, schools are not ashamed to say, "We cannot afford it."

DEVELOPMENTAL RELATIONSHIP-BASED APPROACHES

"Relationship and developmentally focused approaches" is another frequently available category of treatment for ASD. These interventions focus on the social and emotional bonds in children, with the goal being to improve these bonds, often through direct parent involvement. There is less focus on specific behavioral interventions (as in ABA therapy). The intervention is individualized, based on the child's developmental level, regardless of age. The specific treatments falling under this category of interventions are Developmental Individual-Difference Relationship-Based (DIR/Floortime) and the related intervention of The Play and Language for Autistic Youngsters (PLAY) Project. Relationship-development intervention (RDI) also has a similar focus.

In DIR/Floortime, the parent and therapist engage the child on his or her level (on the floor) through activities that the child enjoys. The therapist teaches the parent to engage and direct the child into ever-increasing complex interactions. The focus is on emotional development and the relationship of the parent and the child. This facilitates emotional growth, creativity, relationships, and communication. Two studies in 2011 indicated that this intervention was associated with some improvements in the core symptoms of autism.

The PLAY Project is based upon DIR/Floortime but is designed to train professionals and parents of young children (18 months to 6 years) with autism to provide intense, developmental interventions. In 2014, a study showed that this intervention was associated with improvements in some core symptoms of autism as well as parent and child interactions.

RDI helps the child with ASD to form personal relationships and focuses on thinking flexibly. This therapy also focuses on understanding different perspectives, coping with change, and integrating sensory information.

We do not yet have enough empirical data about these therapies for them to be considered validated treatments, so ABA remains the therapy of choice for many professionals and families (2,7). You may be able to find therapists providing this type of therapy near your home. These therapies can be used alone or in combination with other therapies mentioned in this chapter.

COMPREHENSIVE TREATMENT MODELS FOR EARLY INTERVENTION FOR PRESCHOOL CHILDREN

The Early-Start Denver Model (ESDM) is an early intervention for ASD in preschoolers that is intensive and combines ABA techniques with relationship-based and developmental approaches. This treatment has shown benefits in adaptive, cognitive, and language skills in toddlers with ASD. This approach includes parent training and the involvement of both the therapist and the parent. The emphasis is on parent–child communication. Parents have been found to have "proficient skill" in ESDM techniques by the fifth to sixth hour of treatment. It has been found to provide good outcomes from a clinical and economic perspective. Currently, this is the only validated model for use in children as young as 18 months. It is used in children up to 48 months. Various professionals from different fields can be trained in this model. If you have a very young child with autism and there is a professional trained in this model near you, this would be a great option (2,7).

Learning Experiences and Alternative Program for Pre-Schoolers and their Parents (LEAP) is another early intervention option for children with ASD. It is operated in an inclusion classroom, a general education classroom in which students with and without disabilities learn together. Incidental learning takes place, as well as daily exposure to typically developing children who are trained in skills to aid in improvements of those with ASD in the areas of social skills and communication. This model has been replicated and has shown improvements in IQ and language functioning (7).

PARENT TRAINING

In most treatments or interventions, parents are at least indirectly involved, so in a sense parent training at some level is present in most interventions. There are, however, specific parent training programs for parents of children with ASD. The outcomes have been an increased knowledge about ASD in general as well as appropriate intervention techniques. More recent evaluations of these parent training programs have shown improvements in parent's mental health, better parent–child interactions, improved understanding by parents of their child's difficulties, and improved outcomes on measures of communication and social behavior (2).

There is evidence that a number of specific parent training programs are associated with these improvements in children with ASD. These include the following:

The Autism Spectrum Conditions–Enhancing Nurture and
    Development (ASCEND) parent training program
The Triple P Positive Parenting Program
The Incredible Years Parent Training program adapted for children
    with developmental disabilities

A parent training component added to the early childhood special
  education curriculum
A parent training model for parents of children with ASD introduced in the People's Republic of China.

Also, there is a group-based parent training program
for young children with ASD called Group Intensive Family
Training (GIFT). This group program has shown improvements in adaptive and cognitive functioning of these children.
Stepping Stones Triple P (SSTP) is a structured parenting
program specifically designed for families of children with
ASD that focuses on social learning principles. Recent studies
of this program have shown improvements in parental confidence, increased parent ability to manage and respond to difficult behaviors, and a reduction in child behaviors (7). Lastly,
Parent-Child Interaction Therapy (PCIT) has demonstrated
improvements in child adaptability and shared affect between
parent and child.

It is not important for you to know what each of these programs entails, but you should remember that there are many such
parent training programs available (2).

Although there is some variability among parent training
programs, they should include use of individual sessions and
group sessions, focus on the parents' attainment of knowledge
and skill, and emphasize the need for family support (2).

Overall, parent training has been shown to improve both
knowledge related to ASD and skills to promote more effective
management of behavior. It has been found to reduce stress and
depression, improve parental responsiveness and emotional
regulation, and improve overall parent mental and physical
health (2).

SOCIAL SKILLS GROUPS

The majority of interventions for adolescent children with ASD focus on social skills. Many different social skills interventions have been developed, and they vary widely. The main approaches have been classified as social stories, manualized instructional programs, non-manualized training and support groups, cognitive-behavioral therapy, parent or family mediated, peer mediated, and activity based. Parental involvement in these interventions varies, but most of them at least involve parental assessment before and after the intervention. Social skills programs that include a higher amount of parental involvement include the Junior Detective Training Program, the Program for the Education and Enrichment of Relationship Skills (PEERS), parent-delivered cognitive-behavioral social skills program, and a behavior skills training delivered by the family. One of the difficulties of social skills programs is that children and adolescents have a hard time generalizing the skills to other environments. Family involvement in these programs may help encourage this much-needed generalization (2). Social skills are an important part of any child's treatment plan, and all children should get this therapy. Also, for children and adolescents who are high functioning, this form of therapy may improve their biggest deficit: social skills.

TEACCH PROGRAM

The TEACCH (Treatment and Education of Autistic and Related Communication Handicapped Children) program has been noted to be an evidence-based comprehensive treatment model for children with ASD. The TEACCH program relies on four basic components: physical structure and organization of events, visual information, communication, and specific child interests as rewards.

Unlike LEAP and ESDM (see earlier in the chapter in the section entitled "Comprehensive Treatment Models for Early Intervention for Preschool Children"), this program is for children of all ages and not simply for preschoolers. It focuses on individual strengths and differences, structure, and visual learning; it emphasizes psychoeducation in all environments; and it involves a high degree of collaboration with the family. There is substantial parent involvement; in fact, the parents are often co-therapists. It has been shown that the mother's teaching skills significantly improved with this intervention, and parents often found the program "extremely helpful." They also found it helped them to better manage difficult behaviors (2).

SPEECH THERAPY

Speech therapy is an important part of any treatment regimen for a child with ASD. Children who are nonverbal can be taught to communicate through the use of alternative communication modalities, including sign language, communication boards, picture exchange, visual supports, and programs on tablets. There is evidence to support the use of Picture Exchange Communication System (PECS), sign language, and voice output communication aids. However, even those individuals with ASD with fluent speech need to focus on pragmatic language skills. Thus, most children with ASD need speech therapy. Also, it is doubtful that the amount of speech therapy provided in school is ever sufficient. I recommend a private speech therapy evaluation (outside of school) and regular, private speech therapy sessions unless the private speech therapist states it is not needed (8).

GENERAL RECOMMENDATIONS

Although a treatment plan should always be tailored to your child, I strongly believe that every child with ASD needs at least an initial evaluation with a speech therapist, a physical therapist, an occupational therapist, a child psychiatrist or a developmental pediatrician, and an ABA therapist. If any of these professionals feel that therapy/treatment from their particular field is not needed for your child, then that is good news. However, I would recommend regular follow-up with a developmental pediatrician or a child psychiatrist to ensure that medications are not needed. Your child's needs may change over time, especially if mood symptoms or anxieties develop and need treatment. Also, any child, no matter the age, can benefit from some form of ABA therapy. ABA therapists are the experts in behaviors and catching your child up to his or her peers in a wide range of areas.

One of the biggest issues is not whether your child can benefit from ABA therapy but whether your child has access to this therapy. Often there is not an ABA provider in your area or you cannot afford it because health insurance does not typically pay for this therapy. Call your government representatives to urge them to pass an autism law to mandate ABA therapy coverage by health insurance companies in your state. Some states have passed these laws, but they usually have unreasonable age limits or poor coverage in terms of the number of hours per week allowed. ABA is the most evidence-based treatment for ASD and should be covered! I can attest that ABA therapy has dramatically helped my own daughter.

REFERENCES

1. Mohammadzaheri F, Koegel LK, Rezaee M, Rafiee SM. A randomized clinical trial comparison between Pivotal Response Treatment (PRT)

and structured Applied Behavior Analysis (ABA) intervention for children with autism. *J Autism Dev Disord.* 2014;44(11):2769–2777.

2. Karst JS, Van Hecke AV. Parent and family impact of autism spectrum disorders: a review and proposed model for intervention evaluation. *Clin Child Fam Psychol Rev.* 2012;15:247–277.

3. Reichow B, Barton EE, Boyd BA, Hume K. Early intensive behavioral intervention (EIBI) for young children with autism spectrum disorders (ASD). *Cochrane Database Syst Rev.* 2012;10:CD009260.

4. MacDonald R, Parry-Cruwys D, Dupere S, Ahearn W. Assessing progress and outcome of early intensive behavioral intervention for toddlers with autism. *Res Dev Disabil.* 2014;35:3632–3644.

5. Fava L, Strauss K. Response to early intensive behavioral intervention for autism: an umbrella approach to issues critical to treatment individualization. *Int J Dev Neurosci.* 2014;39:49–58.

6. Grindle CF, Hastings RP, Saville M, et al. Outcomes of a behavioral education model for children with autism in a mainstream school setting. *Behav Mod.* 2012;36(3):298–319.

7. Tonge BJ, Bull K, Brereton A, Wilson R. A review of evidence-based early intervention for behavioural problems in children with autism spectrum disorder: the core components of effective programs, child-focused interventions and comprehensive treatment models. *Curr Opin Psychiatry.* 2014;27:158–165.

8. Volkmar F, Siegel M, Woodbury-Smith M, et al. Practice parameter for the assessment and treatment of children and adolescents with autism spectrum disorder. *J Am Acad Child Adolesc Psychiatry.* 2014;53(2):237–257.

9. Donaldson AL, Stahmer AC. Team collaboration: the use of behavior principles for serving students with ASD. *Lang Speech Hear Serv Sch.* 2014;45(4):261–276.

THE EDUCATIONAL SYSTEM AND
AUTISM SPECTRUM DISORDER

Navigating the educational system is likely the most treacherous and frustrating part of raising a child with autism spectrum disorder (ASD). Often parents feel that they have to be lawyers to understand the rights of their child and to advocate for appropriate resources at school. I know firsthand how difficult this can be. I can honestly state that next to a child's severe tantrums, this is the most frustrating and pervasive problem parents may encounter. Typically, year after year and IEP (individualized education program) meeting after IEP meeting, the battle for even substandard education and services continues.

Parents naturally assume that the school system would have to maintain certain standards and provide appropriate education and therapies for their child. One might even believe that the special education teacher, and the school district itself, would be more expert than the parent. Unfortunately, this is rarely the case. Training, especially specific to ASD, is usually quite poor.

Aside from some very caring teachers, the system is often set up to fail the child.

The school district likely saves money by refusing to provide additional services, modifications, or accommodations for your child. Typically, neither the school district nor the teacher will offer new services or resources to be expended on your child unless it is in their best interest. In most cases, you will have to fight for every resource you can get for your child. Do NOT be passive. Educate yourself about your rights and the possible resources available to your child. Talk to other parents in the autism community about the resources their children are receiving.

Like many parents, I too at first felt that being professional and "nice" was the best way to get my child "good" services. I thought, "You catch more flies with honey than vinegar." Unfortunately, this naiveté did not pay off: things only worsened with this approach. It was not until we learned more about our rights as parents and challenged the school system that things improved at all. It often feels as if the school system equates kindness with weakness and ignorance. Be assertive and do not let the administrators take advantage of your child. Show them that you have certain expectations for your child and the school system. Ask to see their data on your child regarding behaviors and academic work. Ask for accountability and expect it. As a last resort, if all else fails, consider hiring a lawyer or advocate. Sometimes, having a lawyer or advocate at the IEP meeting is all that is needed to spur more appropriate and fair action from the school district.

My perspective comes from being not only a parent of a child with ASD but also a child psychiatrist who has witnessed over a decade of multiple school systems treating children with special needs in a way that should be the headline of newspapers everywhere. Special needs education in America feels like the kind of education that would be seen in a third world country. It is embarrassing and shameful. Furthermore, there is a remarkable

level of deceit and corruption that rivals Washington, D.C. poli-
tics. The level of problems in special education does vary depending on your state and school district, but do not be fooled: there is
likely no "good" school district. Be careful before uprooting yourself and your family to move to what you think is a "better" school
system. The grass is not always greener on the other side.

I have treated many children with ASD who have been
refused IEPs. I am not an attorney, but I strongly feel that all
children with ASD should have an IEP and a behavior intervention plan (BIP). I have even treated nonverbal children whose
parents were told that their child was not eligible for speech
therapy because he or she could not yet speak. They were told
that until the child could speak "some," they would not offer this
service. This is as absurd as it is heartbreaking. All children with
ASD should receive at least an evaluation for speech therapy and
occupational therapy. Also, in the school system speech therapy
is almost exclusively done in a group setting, not individually.
Clearly, the therapy is quite "watered down."

Ideally, children with ASD would also get Applied Behavior
Analysis (ABA) therapy at school (as discussed in Chapter 8).
However, since we cannot even get all states, as of yet, to pass a law
mandating that insurance companies pay for this in the private
sector, it is not likely the school system will do this anytime soon.
It would be expensive as well. However, there should at the very
least be ABA tutors or registered behavior technicians (RBTs) in
every classroom in which there are children with ASD. This is
less expensive than a Board Certified Behavior Analyst (BCBA).
ABA therapists are the experts on behavioral issues associated
with ASD and can manage the behavioral problems more effectively than other school personnel. This would help the classroom
run more smoothly and allow the teacher to teach instead of dealing with behaviors all day long. This would also mandate some
sort of real training for paraprofessionals who deal with ASD.

Ideally, these registered behavioral technicians would replace the paraprofessional or teacher's aide in these classrooms without much (if any) additional cost. Our children would be more likely to be well adjusted and thus would be better able to participate in their education. Additionally, I have had many patients who actually have developed worse behavior with a one-to-one paraprofessional because the paraprofessional inadvertently reinforced bad behavior due to lack of autism training and understanding. This does a disservice to the child and to the school system, which is spending money only to achieve worse outcomes.

Many parents relocate in order to be in the best school district, but this is more complicated when it comes to children with ASD. As a parent, you need to research the special educational services available in the area, especially those related to autism. Certainly the best way to do this is to talk to other parents of children with ASD. An easy way to do this is to contact the nearest autism support group. Also, all children on the autism spectrum are unique, so what may be best for one person's child may not be best for your child. For example, some very high-functioning children may do well in a private school setting with a low student-to-teacher ratio, while others, due to behavioral issues, would be kicked out immediately from the private school and would do better in a self-contained class in public school. Others may do well in a co-taught setting.

Most often private schools are not best for those with ASD because they are not usually tolerant of differences or behavioral problems. Also, they do not feel they have to "put up with" a child's behavior problems, whereas public schools must figure out a way to accommodate your child on some level. On the other hand, public schools try to put your child in the "least restrictive" environment, and this may or may not be best for your child. Be careful not to be flattered if your child is put in a regular education classroom. This is cheaper for the school system. Generally, a regular education classroom is thought to be best for the child since it allows him or her to model typical peer behaviors. However, if the child is disruptive to the class and is not getting the educational assistance needed, then you may not be accomplishing much. The child may be embarrassing himself or herself by odd or aggressive behaviors, causing him or her to be shunned by peers. In this case, the child may not be getting a good education or improvement in social skills. You need to weigh how much your child is learning against better interaction with typical peers.

For this reason, a co-taught classroom can be best. In a co-taught class, a regular education teacher and a special education teacher both teach the same class. Both teachers are responsible for all children in the class, which reduces stigma to the special needs child. With this co-taught model, the child with ASD may get a better education while still being in a class with typical peers. It can be the best of both worlds. However, this is more expensive for the school system than a typical classroom.

It is vital that you have some basic understanding of the educational system and your rights. Remember, you are paying for this school system with your taxes. Also, legally your child has the right to a "free, appropriate public education." Although I am not an expert in educational law, I believe the following information is the most important in dealing with the school system. This is based on my research and experience (personal and professional) over the last decade.

The Individuals with Disabilities Education Act of 1990 (IDEA) was amended in 1997 and again in 2004. This is the law that protects your child's education. One aspect of this federal law is that it emphasizes "child find." This means that every state that receives federal funding under this law has a responsibility to be proactive in finding children in the community who need special education services. They are to "advertise" this availability to parents. It also requires the identification, location, and evaluation of children with disabilities in private schools. However, this does not require that the states provide these specific services in a private school setting (1).

Referrals for special education (IEP) evaluation by the school district can be made by parents, principals, teachers, or mental health professionals. Although referral by a mental health professional does not require a special education assessment, it is difficult for the school district to deny an evaluation as it is the district's responsibility to "child find" or locate children in need of such assessment. You should get your child's psychologist, ABA therapist, and/or psychiatrist to write a letter to the child's school with the child's diagnosis, recommended educational interventions, and any other pertinent information about your child. This can help make sure your child is qualified for special education services and that appropriate modifications are made.

To be eligible for special education or an IEP, your child has to meet certain criteria per the IDEA law. A child with a disability, according to IDEA, "is a child (1) with mental retardation, hearing impairments (including deafness), speech or language impairments, visual impairments (including blindness), serious emotional disturbance, orthopedic impairments, autism, traumatic brain injury, other health impairments, or specific learning disabilities and (2) who, by reason thereof, needs special education related services." Both (1) and (2) criteria must be met; thus, the child must both have a disability and need special education services in order to benefit from education (1).

A child who does not qualify under IDEA for special education (IEP) is still likely to be entitled to some protection under Section 504 of the Rehabilitation Act of 1973, which is typically called a "504 plan" in practice. Section 504 protects individuals with a disability from "discrimination in a major life activity" such as education. Thus, a student with a disability must receive benefits and services comparable to those provided to his or her nondisabled peers. Often children with ADHD who do not meet IDEA criteria for an IEP fit into a 504 plan and can receive some accommodations at school (1).

The first thing to do if you suspect that your child needs special education services is to request, in writing, an evaluation or assessment. You should mail this to your child's school and keep a record of when it was sent. If your child attends a private school or is homeschooled, you should mail it to the school district office. Then the school district is required to develop an assessment plan within a reasonable time period for the parent's approval. The school district must get written parental consent for the plan as well as conduct an evaluation of all areas of suspected disability. A determination of eligibility for special education must be made based on this information and a copy of the report given to the parents (1).

The parent has the right to an independent evaluation at the public's expense if the school district refuses to conduct the evaluation or determines that the child is not eligible. If an assessment tool was used that did not capture all relevant information, this would also be grounds for the independent evaluation. If an evaluation at public expense is requested by the parent, the school district may ask for an administrative hearing. If this happens and the hearing officer determines it should not be done at the public's expense, an independent evaluation at the parent's expense can still be done. The information derived from the independent evaluation must then be considered by the school district when determining the child's eligibility for special education (1).

There are many rules governing the running of an IEP meeting. The parent has a right for the meeting to be scheduled "at a mutually agreed on time and place." If the school district calls you to give you the time of the meeting, you have the right to ask for another time and date. It is vital that the parent(s) be able to make it to the meeting. The parent is an integral and necessary part of the meeting. There is no better advocate for your child than you. Do not be intimidated. You are an equal participant in the meeting, not a bystander. You also have the right to invite anyone who has knowledge or expertise about your child. This could be a professional advocate, psychologist, psychiatrist, ABA therapist, and so forth. If you don't think you can be assertive enough or the best advocate for your child, then hire an advocate or lawyer to help you. Advocates typically charge a reasonable fee and can alleviate some of your stress and the natural confusion that comes along with an IEP meeting.

Although it sounds negative, please understand that not all people at the IEP meeting have your child's best interests at heart. Most of them are representing the school system, and the child's interests and the school district's interests are not necessarily the same, especially when it comes to providing potentially costly resources for your child (1).

At the IEP meeting, the team as a group reviews all evaluations and information. This also includes "consideration of special factors." As an example, for a child whose behavior impedes his or her learning or that of others, the team must come up with appropriate behavioral interventions and supports to address such behavior. The team also considers any "related services" that are needed for the child to benefit from his or her education. In the case of children with ASD, this is usually occupational therapy and speech therapy but might include other therapies. In my opinion, this should also be ABA therapy, but this is unlikely to happen in most school districts due to cost. However, if your child's behavior suddenly worsens, you may be able to ask for an ABA therapist evaluation or "functional analysis" as a temporary measure (1).

When there is agreement among team members, a written document called the IEP is created. This must include statements about the child's current academic performance, measurable goals, specialized instruction, related services, and supports that will be provided. Also, the IEP should include a statement of the extent to which the child will not participate in the mainstream environment or classes, modifications in standardized tests, start date of services, transitional needs (if the child is older than 13), measurable goals, and notification to parents regarding progress (1).

DISCIPLINARY ACTION

The law requires a free and appropriate public education. Thus, issues of discipline can get complicated. A child with an IEP can be punished for the same infractions as other children, but there are certain limits. Children with an IEP can be suspended for no more than 10 consecutive school days per academic year without triggering an IEP meeting. If suspensions of less than 10 consecutive days represent a pattern and add up to more than 10 days, limits will be set. A child with an IEP, similar to other children, can still be placed into an alternative school setting for up to 45 days if the violation involves drugs or weapons (1).

If an IEP is necessary due to the disciplinary action, the IEP team must decide if the behavior was a "manifestation of the child's disability." If it was not a manifestation of the child's disability, then the child may be punished as any other child. If it is a manifestation, then the IEP team must look at the current educational placement to ensure that it is appropriate. For example, if a child's behavior is primarily disruptive, then the team may need to consider more supports. If the child does not already have a BIP, one must be formulated with parents and professionals. This BIP must contain specific areas of concern, how to reduce them, how progress or regression will be assessed and monitored, and the result the team is seeking (1).

If a child is expelled as disciplinary action, the school is still required to provide a free, appropriate public education. Often the school system recommends homeschooling, but parents do not have to agree to this. The school district must always provide education in the least restrictive setting (1).

If the child requires residential treatment to benefit from education, the cost is not to the parents but to the school district. Obviously, this cost is very high and the school district will certainly do this only as a last resort. If parents and the school district disagree, then per IDEA there can be mediation and, lastly, a due process hearing (1).

If the child is incarcerated, the IEP remains intact. The juvenile facility must still provide education consistent with the IEP. Also, mental health services must still be provided, although typically not by the same provider (1).

You must remember that the IEP is your most powerful tool to get the services your child needs and deserves. But if you do not know your rights, you may be steamrolled by the school system. The fewer services that school administrators give your child, the more money the school district gets to keep or use on something else. They save money when you do not know your rights. It is as simple as that.

As proof of school districts' conflict of interest regarding your child's education, please note the following. Since fiscal year 2000, funding has been provided to the states based on whatever level of IDEA funding (or number of IEPs) the state received in 1999. The remainder of the funding is split by the state's share of population (85% of those dollars) and its share of poverty (15%). The states allocate their federal dollars to school districts using the same formula. This creates an incentive for the school district to reduce the number of IEPs given out even if the actual number of cases of ASD or other disabilities is on the rise. Also, even when an IEP is given to a child, certainly there is incentive to provide fewer services for the child to cut costs for the school district.

I know, it is terrible. Recent studies have shown that this system is horribly flawed and can result in certain states or school districts getting 50% more (or less) dollars per child with an IEP than another state or school district. Call your representatives and senators to express your concern about this.

Another problem is that although the IDEA federal law stipulated that the goal was to have the federal government pay 40% of the cost of educating a special needs child, the percentage in reality has never been more than 17%. Typically, the percentage has been about 11%. The rest of the money for special education has had to come from the state and local governments, with the majority coming from the individual states. This is a direct result of Congress cutting funds to education even against its own number of 40% per IDEA.

11 IMPORTANT POINTS FOR INDIVIDUALIZED EDUCATION PROGRAMS

1. Remember that the IEP is a legally binding contract. The school administrators must follow what is written in the IEP. Failure to do so puts them "out of compliance." This gets the state to take notice of the school district if you file a "complaint" that the district is out of compliance. You can do this generally on the school district's website or sometimes by calling a designated number. There is usually a link on the website to the state to file such a complaint. Also, at the IEP meeting, ask for a copy of your rights. The district is required to do so unless you forfeit this.

2. There are five members of an IEP team: the parents, the regular education teacher, the special education teacher, a representative from the school district, and an individual "who can interpret the instructional implications of evaluation results,"

such as a speech therapist or occupational therapist. Members of this team can be excused only if the child's guardian agrees.

3. Remember to put in writing all requests for changes to the IEP or concerns so that the IEP team and school district administrators are held accountable. This may be the most important of all points.

4. As of IDEA 2004, changes to the IEP can take place without an actual IEP meeting if both the parent and the school district agree. I would still recommend that everything be documented or put in writing.

5. The IEP should detail the child's present level of performance. This should contain current information about the child such as strengths and weaknesses, what has worked for the child before, how the child learns best, triggers of behavioral problems, and so forth. This should be based on data from several sources such as parents, teachers, assessments, and other applicable observations.

6. The IEP should contain goals and objectives, with clearly defined criteria. This should include measurable goals with data collection. Educational needs of highest priority should be noted and focused on. The time level for mastery of goals should be 1 year. The goals should explain what the child will do and should describe the condition under which performance is expected (such as with or without prompting or in a small group, etc.). The individual who is responsible for implementing the strategy for goal mastery should be included specifically in the IEP. One way to find out whether the IEP is being followed is to ask to see the data collection on your child.

7. It is important to know the difference between accommodations and modifications in an IEP. They are both supports, but they have different implications. *Accommodations* are allowances in how a child is taught or evaluated but do not change what the child is expected to know. Accommodations may

include extra time, small group learning/setting, large print, and so forth. In contrast, *modifications* change how a child is taught or what is expected of him or her. This can have an impact on diploma options: a child who is not required to meet state curriculum requirements might not get a regular diploma.

8. IEPs have a section called "supports for school personnel." This should include a statement that all staff working with your child with ASD should have special training. It should state, "Staff to be trained in autism teaching strategies" or "staff to be trained in the implementation of the positive behavior intervention plan" for those with BIPs.

9. As the parent, you should prepare for the meeting. Write down important points and concerns so that you do not forget anything. To prove the point you are trying to make, bring as much data as you can, such as your child's papers, recent test grades, handwriting samples, and so forth. Contact a lawyer if you need to understand your rights better. You may even hire an advocate to help you in your IEP meeting. He or she can be with you as an invited guest to the IEP meeting.

10. Under IDEA, parents must always receive prior written notice whenever the school district proposes a change or refuses a request for change of an IEP. This must describe the action being proposed or refused by the school and an explanation of why the proposal or refusal is being made. All data that this decision is based on must be disclosed in writing to the parent.

11. Do not allow the school district administrators to tell you that they cannot provide your child with a service because they cannot afford it or they do "not have the resources." This is not the law. Many of my patients' families are told this, and, sadly, it usually works. It makes the parents feel guilty enough that they back down. Most parents actually accept this as an excuse. Do not allow the school district to do this to you.

PREDICTORS OF YOUR CHILD'S EDUCATIONAL SUCCESS

Based on a National Institutes of Health (NIH) study in 2013, there are important predictors for whether children with ASD will achieve their IEP goals. Although higher IQ, better receptive and expressive language, decreased ASD severity, and increased adaptive behavior all predicted better outcomes for children with IEPs, it was actually child engagement that was more important in predicting outcome. Engagement can be influenced by environmental factors and can possibly be improved regardless of the child's unchangeable characteristics, such as IQ. This study also found that the teacher's experience and the use of evidence-based teaching strategies were unrelated to child outcomes, while teacher burnout was related to fewer improvements. Thus, teachers with more stress and fatigue need more resources and more administrative support. IEP quality was also correlated with child outcomes. Taken together, IEP quality and child engagement accounted for half of the variance in child outcomes, with IEP quality being more important.

Thus, there is real evidence that a high-quality IEP is important in your child's success. And the only way to get a "good" IEP is to know your rights, don't back down, and understand the steps and points mentioned in this chapter (2).

REFERENCES

1. Dalton MA. Education rights and the special needs child. *Child Adolesc Clin North Am.* 2002;11:859–868.
2. Ruble L, McGrew JH. Teacher and child predictors of achieving IEP goals of children with autism. *J Autism Dev Disord.* 2013;43(12):1–24.

10

LONG-TERM PLANNING
AND LEGAL ISSUES

Please be aware that I am not an attorney and the following information should not be considered legal advice. The information contained in this chapter is what I have learned as a parent of a child with autism spectrum disorder (ASD) and as a doctor trying to help those with ASD navigate complex legal and financial decisions. I recommend all parents of children with ASD develop a relationship with a licensed attorney with experience in special needs in their jurisdiction. As this chapter details, there are many different legal issues you and your child may encounter as your child matures into adulthood. Having an attorney who is familiar with your specific situation and your child can be very reassuring should legal needs arise. If you have the financial capacity to place some funds in a retainer with an attorney so that they are available any time you need for a quick e-mail, phone call, or text message, it is often worth the expense and peace of mind. Parents can usually locate attorneys with experience in special needs by contacting their local bar associations, many of which maintain formal referral programs. Also, many autism support groups maintain lists of attorneys who specialize in various aspects of the law relevant to children with ASD. Your child's medical providers may also be able to provide referrals.

FINANCIAL PLANNING

If you are like most parents of a child with ASD, you are overwhelmed with even the thought of long-term planning. You are likely thinking, "It is hard enough making it day by day, let alone considering long-term planning." The truth is that most of us avoid thinking of the future because it is too frightening and uncertain. There is also little guidance from healthcare professionals on this very complex issue. However, much relief can be found in achieving a plan for your child's future. Do not wait.

It is important to talk with a financial planner when your child is young. This will help you be able to plan for your own retirement and financial security, as well as for your child's future. This will also minimize your stress regarding your child's security. How our children will survive when we are gone is a constant nagging thought that looms heavily over us. However, you can prepare for the worst and hope for the best. It is also important to note that all children's trajectories are unique and not very predictable. Thus, in many cases, it is difficult to estimate how much care or support your child will need as an adult until he or she is an adult. Even then, some studies have shown improvements in the 20s, well after transition into adulthood. When your child is young, plan for your child to need life-long care. If your child does not end up needing such care, you and your child will have more money to spend on other important things.

When a person with autism reaches the age of majority (18 years old in most states), you as the parent no longer have the legal rights to which you were entitled throughout your child's youth. You are not able to access your adult child's health or school records, and you cannot make decisions on his or her behalf. For this reason, you will need to consult with an attorney well before your child reaches this age. You and your family (and your child if possible) will need to make some important decisions. These critical decisions are described in the remainder of this chapter.

HEALTH INSURANCE

Health insurance is an important issue to consider. Many adults with ASD need mental health coverage for a variety of psychiatric comorbidities such as depression, anxiety, aggression, attention-deficit/hyperactivity disorder (ADHD), mood instability, and so forth. Furthermore, the medications used to treat your child can be quite costly. Recently, even generics for the treatment of mental health issues have become costly. For these reasons and many more, it is not an option to go without health insurance for your child. If your child has been covered by your private health insurance policy as a child, you must find out what will happen when your child turns 18 or other older ages. This may vary per policy and per state. For example, many insurance policies cover dependents through age 26 or if the adult child is a full-time student. Some may even provide coverage indefinitely for those who are disabled and for whom the parents provide at least 50% of the adult child's support. Other policies may have different stipulations. You must check with your health insurance policy.

Medicaid health benefits are available to those who qualify for Supplemental Security Income (SSI). Adults and children with disabilities who have limited financial resources may also be eligible for Medicaid. Medicaid also provides government funding for long-term services and supports. This can include residential treatment facilities and institutional care in nursing facilities. In my experience, more recently these benefits have been more difficult to obtain even in those who very clearly need it. Do not give up. Keep reapplying or appeal the decision. This greater difficulty is likely secondary to the financial crises of state Medicaid programs. If you believe you meet the income criteria for Medicaid, you may qualify for free legal assistance with your Medicaid denial appeal. This assistance is provided by local affiliates of the federally chartered Legal Services Corporation (LSC). You can visit http://www.lsc.gov to locate your local LSC affiliate.

MEDICAID WAIVER PROGRAMS

The Home and Community-Based Waiver Services "waiver program" is an option available to states to provide "integrated community-based long-term care services and supports to qualified Medicaid recipients." These programs waive some of the rules of Medicaid in order to serve children and adults at home or in the community rather than them requiring an institutional level of care. Since Medicaid is a state program, each state has its own rules about such programs. Thus, you should contact your own state about the specifics of the program in your area. I have found that most parents do not realize these programs exist. The services provided by such programs can remove an enormous weight off the parents' shoulders. For example, some monies can go to provide for sitters, therapists, drivers, vocational rehab, and much more. This also provides much-needed respite care for parents or caregivers. Some states may also require that you apply by a certain age, such as 22 years old, for example. Please do not neglect to research this waiver program (and the age limit to apply by) as it can be quite valuable for your child's future.

GUARDIANSHIP

Parents automatically lose the legal right to make decisions for their child when the child turns the age of majority, even if the child has ASD. Before this age, parents must consider whether guardianship is appropriate and what level of guardianship is necessary. Guardianship is a court-ordered arrangement in which a person is given the legal authority to make decisions for another person who has been declared incapacitated by the court. The following definitions can help you decide what is best for your child.

A *limited guardian* is one who makes decisions in only some specific areas. This is appropriate if your adult child can still make some decisions on his or her own. However, if a guardian is needed for more global decision making, you will need to be a *general guardian*. A *conservator* cannot make any personal decisions but manages the funds of the adult with a disability. If you were the conservator, you could not make medical or other personal decisions, but you would control and manage finances for your child.

Petitions for guardianship or conservatorship must be filed with the appropriate court in the jurisdiction where the child resides, usually based on the county. Guardianship and conservatorship is a lifelong process and the conservator must comply with the court for the lifetime of the individual.

To know how much autonomy your adult child is able to have and how much authority or control you will need, consider how your child makes decisions in important areas. These are generally considered as medical, financial, legal, educational/vocational, living arrangements, safety, self-care, communication, and so forth.

When considering your child's ability to make medical decisions, consider whether he or she can provide accurate information about his or her medical conditions and medications. Can your child weigh the risks and benefits of medical procedures or medications, understand the need for regular medical checkups, know when to get medical help for medical problems, and take a medication that may cause side effects, or allow a painful but necessary procedure?

Consider whether your child understands the purpose of money and is able to count and make change from money. This is important in deciding whether your child can have financial autonomy. He or she must know how to protect his or her money from being stolen, able to budget money, save money for large purchases, and pay bills.

For your child to have authority to make legal decisions, he or she should be able to make sound decisions regarding living arrangements and other major life decisions. Your child should be able to understand the ramifications of signing documents in order to not fall victim to those wanting to take advantage of him or her. Sadly, there are unscrupulous people who not only take advantage of but target adults with special needs.

When determining your child's ability to make decisions regarding education, consider if he or she is able to understand his or her own learning differences and know how to get help or appropriate educational services, such as requesting accommodations from an educational institution. Your child must be able to advocate for himself or herself in the area of education.

For your child to manage his or her own vocational services, he or she must be able to apply for services from the Department of Disability Services and other agencies. Your child will need to be able to access job training or other support services in the area of vocational rehabilitation.

For your child to manage his or her own living arrangements, he or she needs to be able to manage his or her own physical needs such as buying clothes and food, as well as finding reasonable housing. Your child needs to know how to live in a group setting while respecting others' needs for quiet and cleanliness. Your child must also have personal safety skills such as being wary of strangers, avoiding dangerous areas, and keeping doors locked. Your child must be careful and not forgetful around stoves, ovens, or other fire hazards. He or she must know how to call 911 to get help in an emergency and know what constitutes an emergency.

Furthermore, your child needs to be able to communicate his or her own needs. This does not have to be verbally. He or she should be able to understand that he or she has choices and preferences and be able to express these as appropriate.

If your child needs help in any of the areas mentioned, it may be possible to get help for him or her in some areas without requiring guardianship. For example, if your child needs help in making medical decisions, a healthcare agent can be appointed to act on his or her behalf. Also, if your child has difficulty managing finances and receives government benefits, a representative payee can be appointed as part of a conservatorship arrangement or otherwise.

When applying for guardianship, you do not legally need to hire an attorney. However, depending on your family's situation and the number of choices to be made, you may want to consider having an attorney to make the process less painful. An attorney can help you evaluate your options, answer questions about the process, organize your presentation to the court, and serve as emotional support during the court process.

There are several easily accessible resources to get you started in understanding what needs to be done to help secure your child's future. Autism Speaks and www.specialneedsanswers.com are great resources. However, in my opinion most of us are not well equipped to understand the complicated legal and financial decisions that need to be made. Thus, I would recommend finding an attorney who specializes in special needs to make sure everything is done correctly. You certainly do not want any surprises later. A list of such persons can be found on www.specialneedsanswers.com.

SPECIAL NEEDS TRUST

A very important component in preparing for your child's future involves a "special needs trust." This allows you to address the fact that public benefits programs are not sufficient and are often quite inadequate. Also, public benefits programs may change over time, likely becoming more inadequate. Your adult child's needs are likely to change over time as well. Furthermore, having to depend on other family members, especially siblings, to care for your child in the long term can be a significant burden and cause resentment. The special needs trust is the current answer to these problems.

Many times, parents of a special needs child will give their estates to their children not affected by the disability so as to not affect the public benefits of the disabled child. The parents expect that the unaffected children will care for the disabled child. Two important flaws in this are that public benefits are not adequate for the disabled child and rifts in the family may emerge based on unclear expectations of how the unaffected siblings' inheritance should be spent on their disabled sibling.

The special needs trust serves two main functions. First, it manages funds for someone who may not be able to do so due to a disability. Second, it preserves eligibility for public benefits such as Medicaid, SSI, public housing, and other programs.

There are generally two kinds of special needs trusts. A *third-party special needs trust* is created to hold property that is given by someone other than the special needs beneficiary. Anyone can put money into such a trust for a special needs beneficiary, but the person who sets up the trust has the right to decide where the money goes upon the passing of the beneficiary. Second, a *self-settled special needs trust* can be designed to hold property already belonging to the special needs beneficiary. If he or she is a recipient of a state Medicaid program, upon the special needs beneficiary's death, the state program is repaid out of remaining funds from the trust prior to anyone inheriting what is left in the trust.

A trustee, often the custodial parent, manages the trust for the benefit of the special needs beneficiary. The trustee is responsible for ensuring that payments from the trust do not exceed the amounts that would render the beneficiary ineligible to receive public benefits. The trustee must maintain separate bank accounts for funds deposited into the trust and a detailed accounting of all financial activities involving the trust.

The following are important points to consider regarding a special needs trust: no special medical documentation is required; the trust is irrevocable in your child's name once created; the trust owns the assets, not the child; the trust should be separate from any other trust your family may have; and you should hire an attorney to navigate this complicated but important process.

Ensure that any attorney you hire to prepare a special needs trust is licensed to practice in your jurisdiction, is in good standing with your state's bar association, has experience specifically with special needs planning, and carries malpractice insurance.

SSI AND SOCIAL SECURITY DISABILITY INSURANCE/DISABLED ADULT CHILD BENEFITS (SSDI)

Not all children who are in special education will be considered disabled by the Social Security Administration (SSA): in order to do so, they must meet the specific definition of disability and disability-specific criteria set by the SSA. A disability per the SSA is "the inability to engage in any substantial gainful activity by reason of medically determinable physical or mental impairment which can be expected to result in death or has lasted or can be expected to last for a continuous period of not less than 12 months." The disability-specific criteria is set by the SSA in an official publication known as the Bluebook and are divided into adult and childhood sections. The Bluebook is regularly updated, so the best resource is often the SSA website. The Bluebook can be useful in helping parents locate and then highlight the most relevant documentation to support an SSA application.

Two types of benefits are available for people with disabilities over the age of 18: SSI and Social Security Disability Insurance/Disabled Adult Child Benefits (SSDI). The SSA will review documentation and decide whether the person's disability is severe enough and if it prevents the individual from working for a year or more.

Children who have been receiving SSI under the age of 18 will still need to go through a re-determination process to see if they will maintain eligibility of benefits as an adult. This is surprising to many parents. The parent must submit the child or young adult's medical and mental health records, with a list of all hospitals, doctors, facilities, and specialists that the child has seen over the years, to best determine eligibility. The child also will have to have an examination done by a professional paid for by SSA. Unfortunately, this process can take months and sometimes years. For this reason, it is important to start this process as soon as possible.

To be eligible for SSI, an individual must not have greater than $2,000 in countable resources and must have a limited monthly income. Once the child is 18, the income and resources of family members are not counted. This is the case even if the individual lives with his or her parents. The amount of benefits is determined by a number of factors, including any income generated by the person.

SSDI is available to anyone whose disability developed prior to age 22 and whose parent or guardian is either deceased or receiving Social Security retirement or disability benefits. This benefit is available regardless of the person's resources or income.

The SSA will appoint to the disabled person an administrator called a *representative-payee* (rep-payee). This is for all of those who are incapable of managing their own SSI or SSDI benefits. Parents wishing to become the payee for their child's benefits must file an application in person with SSA. A parent can be a rep-payee without having guardianship. Some parents prefer to avoid the more difficult process of guardianship and instead pursue the easier rep-payee process when their child's only income and resources come from Social Security. You must keep careful records of your child's monthly income, and this must be reported to SSA on time. Keep copies of all records sent to SSA.

If your child's application for SSI or SSDI benefits is rejected, or if benefits are reduced, you can take several steps to reverse the decision. There are four levels of the appeals process. Applicants have 60 days to file an appeal at each level of the appeal process. The first step to take if your child's application is rejected is Reconsideration. In this step, you are asking for the case to be reviewed again by the person who originally gave the rejection. The second step is the Appeals Hearing. If your child was denied benefits again during Reconsideration, you can request a hearing before an administrative law judge (ALJ). The ALJ will listen to testimony and review any additional documents that may help prove your case. Applicants have the right to bring a representative to the hearing. The third step is the Appeals Council Review. This is an appeal of the Appeals Hearing/ALJ step. The Appeals Council will review the applicant's file but will not hear new testimony. The fourth and final step is appealing to Federal District Court.

An attorney can help you prepare your child's SSI or SSDI initial application. This is generally recommended because an experienced SSI/SSDI attorney has the best chances of securing SSI/SSDI at the first level. However, prior to any denial by SSA you must pay your own attorney's fees upfront, out of pocket, which is often difficult for families with children of special needs. If your child is denied SSI or SSDI after the Reconsideration stage, then SSA regulations allow you to retain an attorney to prepare your appeal and to have his or her fee paid out of the eventual SSI/SSDI award. The attorney's share of the eventual SSI/SSDI is generally capped at $6,000, or 25% of the SSI/SSDI award. Ensure that any attorney you hire to prepare your child's SSI/SSDI application or appeal is licensed to practice in your jurisdiction, is in good standing with your state's bar association, has experience before the SSA, and carries malpractice insurance.

In lieu of an attorney, the SSA also allows representatives who have passed an SSA exam to represent parties before the SSA. This may be a less expensive option for preparing your child's initial SSI/SSDI application. If you are considering hiring an SSI/SSDI representative who is not an attorney, ensure that he or she is properly authorized to practice before the SSA, is trustworthy, has sufficient experience and training, and is an active member of National Organization of Social Security Claimants' Representatives (NOSSCR) or the National Association of Disability Representatives (NADR). Both of these organizations maintain lists of accredited members on their websites.

From time to time unlicensed fly-by-night SSI/SSDI representatives take advantage of families with children with special needs, make huge promises, demand large upfront fees, and then skip town. Often there is little that can be done in these circumstances to recoup the large fees paid by families, who usually are left at square one regarding their SSA application.

OTHER LEGAL ISSUES

There are other, somewhat more minor legal issues to consider. You and your child must consider whether or not to obtain a driver's license. Discuss with your child's doctor whether or not this is possible or appropriate. You may wish to use a driver's training program. Some technical colleges offer driving training programs, and these programs are required to provide reasonable accommodations for your child's disability under federal law. If your child has problems with focus and this is a concern, you might want to consider a stimulant medication, at least for driving. Also, all males, regardless of disability, must register for Selective Service at age 18. Furthermore, you and your child will need to consider whether or not to register to vote.

LETTER OF INTENT

It is generally recommended that you, as the parent or guardian of a child with ASD, write a letter of intent describing your child. Since you know your child best, you can relate your child's history (medical and otherwise), his or her current status, likes and dislikes, and your hopes for your child's future. You should write this letter immediately and update it as your child's needs change. In this way, should you become disabled or incapacitated, other family members or caregivers can carry out your wishes and learn from your invaluable insights. Although this is not a legal document, it can be helpful as a guide to the court and family members during important considerations.

COMMON MISTAKES TO AVOID

Special needs families must avoid several common mistakes.

Often parents forget that it is beneficiary designations and not their will that determine where their money from bank accounts, individual retirement accounts (IRAs), life insurance, and other financial accounts goes. Furthermore, if you do not designate money to the special needs trust instead of the special needs individual, it will likely hurt your child by making him or her ineligible for public benefits.

Many parents purchase term life insurance to fund a special needs trust as it is more cost-effective in the short run for families. However, permanent life insurance (i.e., universal life, whole life, or variable life) can be more cost-effective over the lifetime of the parents.

Often special needs trusts are drafted into the parents' estate plans to be implemented upon the death of the second parent. However, the trust should be set up before the death and before any gift is made to prevent any loss or delay of public benefits. The trust should be a stand-alone that is immediately operable.

Creating a traditional 529 plan or college savings plan could have disastrous effects for special needs children if they are not going to go to college and need to start receiving public benefits after age 18. Currently SSA counts 529 plan holdings toward the applicant's $2,000 maximum assets cap, so this can disqualify your child from receiving SSI. Some state programs also consider 529 accounts as assets that can disqualify your child from receiving benefits, although many states have begun exempting 529 plans from SNAP and Medicaid.

In lieu of a traditional 529, parents of children with ASD should investigate a 529A plan. 529A plans were created in 2014 to allow families to save for a special needs member without risking eligibility for public benefits. 529A plans can be used to pay for medical co-pays, medical equipment, therapy, and other necessary medical expenses. Like traditional 529 plans, contributions to 529A plans through state-designated financial institutions can be tax-exempt but have their own contribution limits. 529A plans are also excluded from the asset tests in SSI and should be exempt from state-level program asset tests. Many people believe that in time 529A plans may be a replacement for special needs trusts. However, as of this writing, federal and state agencies are still in the process of implementing 529A regulations and few financial institutions offer them. You will want to discuss a 529A with your financial planner or attorney. If you have a young child, it could be something you revisit in two to three years once 529A plans are fully implemented.

Failure to communicate your plans for your child to other family members can cause many problems. Your intentions for your child should be well known to all. Furthermore, the existence of the special needs trust needs to be communicated to all in the family, especially grandparents, because if they make a gift to the child directly, the child may be disqualified from public benefits.

The same person should not necessarily be designated as the executor, guardian, and trustee. The same person you trust to make financial decisions may not be the best caregiver for your special needs child. If you feel there is not a best person for this in your family, there are some agencies that can provide this service.

Be careful not to hire a biased or inexperienced financial planner. This can cost you dearly in the future. Financial planners often work on commission and are treated as salespeople under the law, and they may be tempted to sell you financial products that carry higher hidden fees. I recommend seeking out an independent financial planner to whom you pay a flat fee or an hourly rate for advice regardless of what financial products you invest in. This not only ensures you are getting the best and most impartial advice but can save you and your child's assets tens of thousands of dollars in fees as your child grows older. I also recommend seeking a financial planner who can show that he or she has experience in special needs planning in order to avoid mistakes that could cost your child eligibility for government benefits. Any financial planner you retain should be licensed, insured, and accredited by a reputable agency or professional association.

The earlier you get started on these legal issues, the earlier you can worry less about your child's future. I know that you will want to delay in dealing with the issues in this chapter, but please do not wait. If you are confused about how best to handle your child/family's specific financial or legal situation, hire an attorney and/or a special needs financial planner. Also, do not reinvent the wheel. Reach out to other families that have gone through similar processes. For example, navigating the Medicaid waiver process is laborious, and other families may be able to give you advice. In some communities, there are people who charge a fee to help you with the complex paperwork for the Medicaid waiver. Contact your local autism support group or state resource center. They may be able to advise you or direct you to those who can help you.

YOUR ADULT CHILD AND VOCATIONAL ISSUES

Our main goal as parents of a child with ASD is to help our child achieve his or her greatest potential and highest level of functioning. We also want our child to be well cared for even when we are no longer physically able or after our death. There are ways to ensure that your child is successful in his or her transition into adulthood.

First, make sure that the goals you have for your child are reasonable. Get feedback from your child's providers on his or her level of functioning and potential expectations. But be careful: no one can accurately and definitively predict your child's future level of functioning. Get this feedback in your child's early teens. You want to hope for the best but plan for the worst.

As there is a wide spectrum of levels of functioning among those with ASD, no writer can discuss all the options available to your child. However, if you feel that your child is on a college track, then pursue this. There are many options available, such as regular college, online college, or even special needs programs at various colleges. If you feel that your child has limited ability to work, then apply for disability and get him or her involved in vocational training. Vocational training should start in high school for your child and should be mentioned in a transition plan within an individualized education plan (IEP) when your child is 16 years old. This transition plan focuses on what needs to be accomplished to assist your child in meeting his or her post–high school goals. There are likely many companies in your community that participate in vocational rehab programs. The school system is usually aware of these programs and will help your child participate in them.

If it is clear that your child will need a caregiver indefinitely as an adult, you should pursue the Medicaid waiver program in your state. This allows additional monies to be available for your child. This will assist your child in attending vocational rehab (if applicable) and provide a sitter for your child if needed. Your child will be more independent as he or she will have additional providers in the home to help. Many times my patients on the Medicaid waiver program enjoy feeling less dependent upon their parents. It also gives parents some respite and provides solace that their child has more financial security. Make sure you apply as soon as your child is an adult, or sooner if this is possible in your state. At least some states have deadlines by which you must apply or your child will no longer be eligible. For example, in Georgia, if you do not apply for the Medicaid waiver by age 22, you can never receive this benefit.

Every state is likely to have varying levels of support for adults with ASD. In some states, Medicaid waivers are more helpful than others and with more coverage, such as for Applied Behavior Analysis therapy) (see Chapter 8). Also, adult daycare programs are available in some areas. Some local areas have great options in terms of group homes, should this be needed for your child. An interesting point is that often parents expect their adult child to be living with them until they die. This may not necessarily be best. It is likely better for you to help them transition to a group home or other placement before something happens to you. It is going to be difficult enough for your child to handle your passing without him or her having to handle leaving home and going to a new placement as well. Also, you are the one best suited to find the most appropriate place for your child. You know your child best.

The transition to adulthood can be hard for both the person with ASD and the parent. You will get through it, but make sure you are educated on the above issues. Some information is not well known but is vital to a smooth transition. Do not forget to ask your local autism support group for help with resources and other information during this transition. The Autism Speaks website can be a valuable resource as well.

_____

STAGES OF GRIEF, SPIRITUALITY, AND RELIGION

Dealing with any great stressor challenges our core beliefs about ourselves and about life in general. Most of us have certain reasonable expectations of how things will go in our lives. We will graduate from high school, maybe go to college, probably get married, likely have children, and so on. Small wobbles from our intended path in life are understandable to us. Although we all have different tolerances for frustration in dealing with obstacles in our way, we usually handle these troubles well. None of us expects that tragedy will strike. We never think during pregnancy that our child may have a disability or even that our child could die. We have typical expectations for our child's life similar to those of our own lives.

Thus, when we finally are told that our child has autism, our world comes crashing down. Our worldview is shattered. The plans we had made for our child's life and our futures are forever changed in an instant. The way we cope with this immense challenge changes everything, for us and our child.

At some point during any discussion of autism, we must bring spirituality and religion into the conversation. It is impossible not to do so. Any parent whose child has received the autism diagnosis knows this to be true. This is because in order to cope and find acceptance, we must find meaning. How can we accept this news without adjusting our worldview or understanding of life? We must come to terms with the questions that inevitably arise, such as "Why me?", "How could this happen?", "Whose fault is this?", "What did I do wrong?" Other questions that come to mind for those who already believe in a higher power are "Why would God let this happen?", "Why did God do this to me?", "Am I being punished?", "Why would God allow such suffering, especially for a child?" Sometimes it is only through great trials that we realize the need to find deeper meaning. It is in our darkest moments that we realize that we needed answers to questions we did not know existed. It is then we realize that we did not understand about life what we thought we understood.

When you hear the news that your child has autism spectrum disorder (ASD), the grieving process starts immediately. The child is not dead, but the life you had dreamed of for him or her is dead. You realize that your life will never be the same, but even you cannot imagine just how true this will be. The whole family goes through a slow and prolonged, life-long grieving process. Some have described this as "chronic sorrow." Possibly the worst part is that there is never a clear prognosis for your child's abilities, so there is no way to come to accept a specific degree of disability. As behavioral problems wax and wane, so do the parents' predictions for the future. As it is human nature to do, you fear the worst possible outcome. You are left feeling like you have to wait for decades to know the big picture of what needs to be accepted. This is incredibly painful and overwhelming.

Perhaps even worse, occasionally professionals inappropriately make initial predictions for the child's life that they cannot possibly predict, removing all hope from the parent for more positive outcomes.

Raising a child with autism is a roller coaster of ups and downs. Your child has improvements and then setbacks, or even periods of stagnation. He or she may vacillate between periods of progress and regression. Children with ASD typically have unpredictable, severe tantrums. This causes the parents to be unable to predict the child's future or even their own. During moments of progress the parent feels exceedingly grateful and hopeful. In times of worsened behavior, the parent may feel despair. Given that there is no known cause of autism, a foreseeable cure, or "answers" from professionals, parents are left feeling alone and often helpless and hopeless. Families and friends often retreat because they do not know how to help, and they are offended by the child's behavior. Eventually, most families become isolated. The whole family feels punished. The child's behaviors (especially tantrums) are often so severe that going out in public as a family is a humiliating and at times torturous experience, filled with judging stares from other parents. The child essentially trains the family not to leave home. This furthers the isolation and the feeling that the whole family's life is "abnormal."

Parents have no choice but to feel dragged down and punished, or to rise above the autism and find meaning. In my opinion, the best way to find meaning is to fight the autism and to help others. I love my child for her uniqueness, and I recognize the cute and funny things she does. But I do not specifically love the autism. Thus, I fight ASD as a physician by helping to decrease in my patients as many of the disabling symptoms as I can. I also help my own child as a parent by providing her with medication and as many therapies as possible.

However, you do not have to be a doctor to fight the negative aspects of ASD. You can be an advocate for your child and others with autism. You can be an advocate in your local school district or at the state or federal level. You can join or form a support group, or even be a friend to another parent who is struggling. Helping others makes you feel more grateful for what you do have. It gives you a better perspective and a lot of satisfaction. It provides you with meaning.

I believe that navigating life without religious beliefs is more difficult and painful. This is all the more true when you are dealing with the immense, daily struggle of caring for a child with autism. Religion offers hope. It offers meaning. Without these, you are at a greater risk for depression and despair. You must also not have the perception that God is a vengeful, cruel God who is punishing you by placing autism in your life. This would only add to the shame and sorrow. I am not a theologian, but I state the following because I believe those caring for children with ASD need to hear it. I believe that God will bless those who have suffered so much, especially for caring for innocent children who cannot care for themselves. I believe that if I respect those caregivers of children with autism, how much more must God respect and care about them? I believe that however painful autism may be, God can turn something terrible into something great. He can make beauty out of suffering. You did not do anything to deserve autism. Even scientifically, this appears to be true. You did not cause your child's ASD. I strongly believe that finding faith can help you to heal and find a place of peace and acceptance.

One of the most amazing things about ASD is what it can bring out in other people. I have been fortunate, given my profession, to see very large numbers of the autism community. I have observed that parents or caregivers of these children are some of the most incredible people that you could hope to meet. They are self-sacrificing and would literally do anything for their children.

They love more unconditionally than the parents of any other group of children that I have encountered. They love their children regardless of whether the child reciprocates this love in any outward way. I have tremendous respect for the caregivers of children with autism. Their perseverance is unmatched, especially given the limited resources and support available. They have to fight the world for their child on a daily basis, sometimes getting hit or harmed by the child they are trying to protect. This is truly the silver lining of autism and a reflection of what is best about humanity.

You not have to understand why your child has autism, but simply accept that he or she does. It is a difficult feat, but well worth it. Many times a parent's denial prevents the appropriate and timely treatment with medications and therapies. These delays are harmful to the child and affect his or her later outcome and degree of disability. The parent can easily end up in a situation in which his or her denial hurts the child in that moment and potentially in the future. Unfortunately, I see this very often in my practice and in the autism community.

It is very important for us to understand the grieving process. The most famous model of grief is that given to us in 1969 by Elisabeth Kübler-Ross. It is known as the five stages of grief: denial, anger, bargaining, depression, and acceptance. These stages were originally identified in those dealing with imminent death and not the many other difficult life events to which they have since been inappropriately applied. The theory does not work well in the context of many grief situations. The acceptance stage has since been understood to be more complicated and longer lasting than first proposed by Kübler-Ross. More recently grief experts have moved away from the traditional stage of acceptance to "establishing lasting changes in the worldview after a loss or searching for meaning in a loss as strategies for successful grieving" (1).

Many first-hand accounts describe various emotions related to having a child with a disability, such s: numbness, disappointment, isolation, withdrawal, defensiveness, protest, anger, sadness, despair, shock, denial, self-doubt, humiliation, confusion, disbelief, and guilt. The caregiver may feel hopeless, and this feeling can be perpetuated by friends, family, or healthcare professionals. At times, just when the caregiver may have moments of some peace or less pain, their feelings of grief may be reactivated by a random trigger. This reactivation of grief will happen periodically for the caregiver throughout the child's life and has been termed "chronic sorrow." The grief is especially common during typical life transitions. In a study of mothers of children with a disability, it was noted that the mothers felt sad and wanted to remove the child's disability but also felt content with their child for who he or she was.

This paradox illuminates the fact that the grief process is unique for parents of children with autism: often their happiness coexists with chronic sorrow. I can attest to this very strange feeling. I too want to rid my child of the ASD and her disability, but I also love her "Gabbyisms." I love what makes her who she is at the same time (1).

MEANING-MAKING THEORY OF GRIEF

An interesting grief theory that is more appropriate for parents of children with disabilities and well suited to parents of children with ASD is the "meaning-making" theory of bereavement. This newer theory reportedly came from the assertion made by Viktor Frankl, a Holocaust death camp survivor, that finding meaning in suffering helps us to cope. This theory has been further developed within the last 10 to 15 years.

This theory is rooted in a constructivist perspective. It is thought that we need to "construct and maintain an understanding of ourselves through our experiences and the stories we tell about our experiences." Loss of a loved one or of what we thought our child would be is seen to challenge our understanding of the world and of ourselves. We must then either fit the implications of the loss into our previous understanding of the world and of ourselves, maintaining the consistency of our identity and the way we see life, or we must create a new narrative and understanding. These are the only two options. If we choose the latter way, we must reorganize or expand our beliefs so that the loss will logically fit with our new understanding of the world and of ourselves. The meaning-making process is highly individual, as each person has his or her own religious beliefs, educational background, cultural influences, family dynamics, intrapersonal characteristics, and so on. To make sense out of the loss or make meaning out of it, we must fit the loss into our current spiritual system or change our spiritual system in response to the loss. I believe it is when we are challenged that we realize that our previous spiritual system had many holes in it or was "wrong." It was as if our struggle was inevitable and just waiting for the right stressor to occur (1).

As mentioned in Chapter 3, social support for caregivers of children with ASD is vital for both the caregiver and the child's health and success. The value of social support cannot be overstated. Social support can be formal, such as that provided by community or government agencies, or informal, such as that provided by friends and family. Interestingly, informal support has been shown to be more effective in reducing stress. Studies have shown that mothers of children with ASD first turn to their spouse, then to immediate family, and finally to other parents of children with disabilities. Such support is helpful in the parents' adaptation and in the mental health of the parents and the child. Those with higher levels of support report lower levels of depression-related physical symptoms and fewer marital problems (2).

Another very important type of social support is derived from spiritual or religious sources. According to some studies, greater than 90% of people in the United States believe in God. The degree to which this resource is helpful depends upon the individual's specific religious beliefs and the roles these beliefs serve in his or her daily life. Many studies note that spirituality and religion affect physical and psychological health. Religious affiliation is associated with lower death rates and fewer depressive symptoms. A study found that students who were both spiritual and religious had more "immunity" to stressful situations than those who were spiritual but not religious (2).

Religious beliefs are a set of ideas and values concerning a person's relationship with God and religious community. Religious activities refer to a person's involvement in specific organizational or non-organizational events. These might be attending church services or devotional reading. Spirituality refers to finding meaning from life experiences and may not necessarily be related to the belief in a higher power. Defining these constructs is necessary in discovering which part(s) of religion and spirituality is most important or helpful for the caregiver. For example, one study found that "lower levels of involvement in religious activities were associated with lower levels of depressed affect, whereas higher levels of spirituality were associated with greater prosocial behavior" (2).

Unfortunately, few studies have examined the role of religion and its impact on families affected by ASD. According to one study, only 5% of families of children with ASD stated that they would turn to a member of their congregation for help, while 66% reported they would likely express their personal beliefs in private prayer. Support from these personal beliefs and prayer was related to better health outcomes. In one study, positive religious coping was defined as "seeking a positive relationship with God and experiencing closeness and harmony with God." This type of coping is associated with improvements in social relationships and personal resources. However, negative religious coping was defined as "blaming God or believing that God had abandoned or punished them." This negative type of coping was associated with more depression and anxiety (2).

An important study in 2009 sought to examine religion and break it down into the three constructs of religious beliefs, religious activities, and spirituality. The researchers focused on how these individual parts of religion impacted the outcomes for mothers of children with ASD. The results were very interesting. Both religious beliefs and spirituality were associated with fewer negative and more positive social and emotional outcomes. Both of these constructs were associated with less negative affect of the mother, better parenting affect, and less depression. However, religious activities were associated with more negative and less positive outcomes. Only religious beliefs were related specifically to the level of maternal depression, while only spirituality predicted parenting affect. It may be that the belief in God and the feelings of closeness with God help to counteract the feelings of depression and isolation experienced by mothers of children with ASD. Intuitively, this makes sense. The finding of meaning in life and of autism (greater spirituality) would then relate to more joy in parenting or "parenting affect."

Religious beliefs and spirituality were associated with higher self-esteem, positive life events, life satisfaction, positive affect, optimism, internal locus of control, and psychological well-being. However, only religious beliefs predicted optimism. Religious beliefs and spirituality do not only protect against negative outcomes but also promote positive ones. Mothers who scored higher on measures of spirituality and religious beliefs spent more time focusing on what is really important to them in life (or the meaning of life) and less time on the disability of their child.

Sadly, in the study, involvement in religious activities caused more parenting stress, worsened parenting affect, and depression. The greater the religious activity involvement, the worse was the outcome. Furthermore, involvement in religious activities was associated with lower self-esteem, less positive maternal affect, and worse overall well-being. On the surface, this may be hard to believe. But as a parent of a child with ASD, I understand. It is highly stressful to take a child with ASD into a religious setting. The child can be highly disruptive, and churches are often ill equipped to deal with behavioral problems. This makes attending services painful and certainly not satisfying or supportive. As a parent, you are worrying the whole time about the child's behavior even if he or she is not misbehaving because tantrums are unpredictable. Thus, going to a religious service with a child with ASD is typically not a positive experience.

In conclusion, as a parent of a child with ASD, you should understand that the grieving process can be quite prolonged and even last a lifetime. Please understand that this is "normal." However, it does get better. The grief may last a lifetime on some level, but acceptance does come as well. Instead of ASD always being bitter, it becomes bittersweet. You will learn to find meaning in the struggle and hopefully develop lifelong friendships with those who also understand your struggles. You should also be aware that religion and spirituality together are very important in reducing your level of stress, as well as improving your overall mood and life satisfaction. Although spirituality helps, it is the combination of spirituality and religion that offers the most benefit. If you do not currently have specific religious beliefs, you should pursue them.

RELIGION IN THE INDIVIDUAL WITH ASD

The religious experience of the person with ASD is also complicated. This is an important topic for parents who are religious and want their child to have a personal relationship with God. Discovering religion and spirituality may also be a valuable way for the person with ASD to find meaning, cope with inherent stressors, and find comfort through a relationship with God. Many parents want to know if there are limitations in the understanding of religion or God for an individual with ASD. There is very limited research on this, but I will present what is known so far.

In 2012, a Dutch study that found the more autistic traits an adult had, whether or not they had an ASD diagnosis, the greater was their fear of God and the less positive were their feelings. This is postulated to be related to impairments in social reciprocity and abstract imagination (3).

Mentalizing, or theory of mind, describes our natural ability to understand the mental state of ourselves and others. This underlies overt behavior. Mentalization is an imaginative mental activity that allows us to perceive and interpret human behavior in terms of intentional mental states. This is how we can understand other people's emotions, behaviors, and intentions. Unfortunately, this ability is impaired to varying degrees in those with ASD. This likely undermines the ability to believe in God and understand His intentions, motives, feelings, and behaviors, just as it is for the person with ASD to understand these things in other humans. It may be that mentalizing deficits constrain belief in God (4).

Neuroimaging studies show that thinking about and praying to God activates certain areas of the brain known to be involved in mentalizing abilities. Mentalizing is deficient in those with ASD. Much evidence indicates that mentally representing supernatural beings or God requires mentalizing. In general, men are more likely to score higher for ASD symptoms and more likely to be nonbelievers. Adults with an ASD diagnosis are more likely than others to identify as atheist and are less likely to belong to an organized religion (4).

The results of a study investigating the effect of mentalizing on belief in God in those with ASD are intriguing and informative. The study showed that adults with ASD were only 11% as likely as neuro-typical adults (those without ASD) to strongly endorse God. This was unrelated to IQ. For each standard deviation increase in autism scores, the likelihood of strongly endorsing God dropped by 66%, even after controlling for gender. In a separate but related study, higher autism scores in those without an ASD diagnosis again predicted lower belief in God. It was found that mentalizing mediated this effect. In adults without ASD, men were lower in mentalizing than women and, as a result, had a lower belief in God: men were only 60% as likely to report strong belief in God (4).

Therefore, it may be much more difficult for those with ASD to understand God or to have a traditional relationship with God. However, I do believe this depends upon the individual, because each person with ASD has unique deficits and abilities. I have known many with ASD who do have an understanding of God, but it may be more rigid or more "black and white" than a typical peer. Please do not take this to mean that children with ASD are incapable of learning about God. I teach my own child about God, and she very much loves it. However, you will need to be more careful about what you teach your child and how he or she is understanding what you are teaching. Remember that these children are often quite literal and concrete. For example, if you tell your child that God will answer his or her prayer, the child may expect the wish to be granted, and right away.

REFERENCES

1. Douglas HA. Promoting meaning-making to help our patients grieve: an exemplar for genetic counselors and other health care professionals. *J Gen Couns.* 2014;23(5):695–700.
2. Ekas NV, Whitman TL, Shivers C. Religiosity, spirituality, and socio-emotional functioning in mothers of children with autism spectrum disorder. *J Autism Dev Disord.* 2009;39:706–719.
3. Schaap-Jonker H, van Schothorst-van Roekel J, Sizoo B. The God image in relation to autistic traits and religious denomination. *Tijdschrift voor Psychiatrie.* 2012;54(5):419–428.
4. Norenzayan A, Gervais WM, Trzesniewski KH. Mentalizing deficits constrain belief in a personal God. *PLoS One.* 2012;7(5):e36880.

12

———

NAVIGATING THE JOURNEY

Following the recommendations and using the knowledge in this book will help you to navigate your journey successfully. Your child will make progress and you will value and enjoy every new milestone. You will experience unconditional love and patience. You will have great joy in your life. You will love your child for his or her unique personality and perspective on life. Your child is different, but not "less." Embracing your child's differences will open your heart and mind to new possibilities and pathways.

If your child has not been diagnosed officially yet, you must have your child evaluated as soon as possible. Early diagnosis and treatment will help to significantly improve your child's prognosis and future. You must understand the negative effects of your child's autism on your whole family and how to avoid them as much as possible. Surround yourself with people who "get you" and your family. You need support. Fight the urge to isolate yourself and your family. Create and maintain a healthy marriage. Explore all treatment avenues, such as medications, therapies, and complementary and alternative medicine (CAM) treatments as appropriate. Do not be afraid to consider medications. Find a provider you trust who is an expert with ASD.

For your child to be successful, you need to become very familiar with the educational system and be an advocate for your child at school. You also need to be adept with legal issues of guardianship and other long-term planning issues such as the special needs trust.

Lastly, you need to find acceptance and may need to explore issues of spirituality and religion.

Since my daughter's diagnosis 10 years ago, I have found great joy in raising her. I appreciate and love her for who she is every day. My family would not be complete without her. Not a day goes by that she does not make me laugh. She has given my life great purpose and fulfillment, and I have no doubt that you feel the same about your child. I am amazed at the progress she has made. My expectations were dim after she was first diagnosed, but her progress has left me in awe of the strength and determination she has displayed. She has broken through barriers I had not expected her to surpass.

Michael A. Ellis, DO, graduated from Nova Southeastern University College of Osteopathic Medicine with a Doctor of Osteopathic Medicine degree in 2004, with highest honors. He completed his General Psychiatry residency program and Child and Adolescent Psychiatry fellowship (2009) at the Medical College of Georgia. He is a Clinical Assistant Professor at Mercer University School of Medicine, Clinical Associate Professor at the Philadelphia College of Osteopathic Medicine, GA Campus, and Clinical Assistant Professor at the Medical College of Georgia. He is also the Medical Director of Child and Adolescent Psychiatry at The Bradley Center. He has been a member of the American Academy of Child and Adolescent Psychiatry (AACAP) Work Group on Life Long Learning from 2009 to the present.

Dr. Ellis has a wife and three children. His oldest child has autism spectrum disorder (ASD). After the family settled in the community of Columbus, GA, parents brought their children to see him both because ASD is within his scope of practice and because they correctly assumed that having a daughter with autism afforded him a unique perspective when treating other children on the autism spectrum. He decided to write this book as a guide for parents that includes what he wishes he had known when his daughter was diagnosed and what he believes you and your family will need to know about living with autism.

Index

References to tables are indicated with an italicized *t*.